Unveiling Maternal Health Care Realities in Arunachal Pradesh

Unveiling Maternal Health Care Realities in Arunachal Pradesh

A Case Study of Mebo Sub-Division

Dr Apilang Apum

KALPAZ

Published by

Kalpaz Publications
C-30, Satyawati Nagar,
Delhi – 110052
Ph.: 011-47034999, 9811692060
www.kalpazpublications.com
E-mail: kalpaz@hotmail.com

Distribution Network
www.gyanbooks.com
India, USA, Canada, UK, Australia, France

ISBN: 978-93-5722-567-0 (PB)

First Published, 2025

Printed at: Gyan Press, Delhi.

Unveiling Maternal Health Care Realities in Arunachal Pradesh
Author: DR APILANG APUM

To my beloved father, *Late Shri Bapok Apum*, and my mother, *Mrs. Toti Megu Apum*—whose unwavering love and guiding wisdom have been the pillar of strength throughout my academic journey. Their sacrifices and encouragement have shaped every step of my path, and this work stands as a humble tribute to their enduring presence in my life.

Contents

Preface

This book is the culmination of both academic inquiry and heartfelt dedication. It stems from my dissertation work submitted to Rajiv Gandhi University, Rono Hills, Doimukh, Itanagar as part of the Master of Philosophy in Economics, and explores a topic of profound social importance—**The Status of Maternal Health Care Utilisation in Mebo Sub-Division, East Siang District, Arunachal Pradesh.**

Maternal health lies at the intersection of public health, gender equity, and human development. Yet in rural areas, particularly those nestled within challenging geographical terrains, access remains uneven. This study not only investigates the status and patterns of maternal health care services—such as antenatal care, institutional delivery, and postnatal support—but also delves into the underlying factors and socio-cultural barriers that shape their utilisation.

The research combines both statistical analysis and lived experiences, aiming to offer insight and practical reflections that may inform future policy efforts. My hope is that this work contributes meaningfully to ongoing dialogues around improving maternal health services, particularly in underserved tribal regions.

I humbly dedicate this book to my beloved Father Late Shri Bapok Apum and Mother, Mrs. Toti Megu Apum, whose love and guidance have been my enduring strength. My academic journey has been deeply enriched by the faculty of Rajiv Gandhi University, Itanagar and supported by friends, family, and respondents who shared their stories.

Above all, I acknowledge the grace of God for offering me the clarity and resilience to pursue this research with purpose and compassion.

Chapter - I

Introduction

Health is a state of complete physical, mental and social wellbeing and not merely the absence of disease or infirmity[1]. The WHO 1978 declaration amplified it to include the ability to lead a "socially and economically productive life"[2] Health is considered as a fundamental human right and a basic need for an improved quality of life. The United Nations Organisation in 1979, adopted health as an integral part of socio-economic development and not only a part of scientific study. As health occupies important space in development paradigm, it is integral to economics too. Good health and better access to health service adds to productivity through both psychological (motivation) and physical (labour) aspects. This may cumulate to increase in their income and standard of living which further help in growth of economy.

A nation's growth is therefore not just about tallying agricultural, industrial and service balance sheets but also about the quality of Human Development. Considering this aspect the governments across the globe are trying to achieve better health standards as well as to provide accessible health care services.

1.1 Evolution of Health Economics

After World War II, the health sector experienced high levels of expansion, rationalisation and organisation. In the late 1950s and

1. WHO 1948
2. WHO, 1978, declaration of Alma-Ata: health for all series no. 1, http//www.who.int/en/

by the beginning of 1960s economics began its incursion to health issues. Selma Muskin one amongst health economist defines health economics as a broader science that is concerned with the optimum use of scarce economics resources for the care of the sick and the promotion of health taking into account competing uses of these resources. Considering health as investment she argued that people develop themselves by investing in health services and education with a future return associated with it (Selma Muskin, 1958).

Similarly Grossman (1972) considered health as a stock which degrades overtime in the absence of investment and therefore health was viewed as a capital. Each individual is both a producer and a consumer of different types of healthcare service. As a consumption good, it yields direct satisfaction and utility and as an investment it yields satisfaction to the consumer indirectly through increased productivity, fewer sick days and thereof, higher wages. Economist have pointed out that good health gives good income in the labour market. World development report (1993) explains good health as a crucial to wellbeing. Spending on it can be justified purely on economic grounds. Health economics is, therefore, broadly "the application of the theories, concepts and techniques of economics to the health sector". It is, concerned with such matters as the allocation of resources between various health promoting activities, the quantity of resources used in health services delivery; the organisation and funding of health service institutions, the efficiency with which resources are allocated and the effects of preventive, curative and rehabilitative health services on individuals and society. Thus, health economics is the application of the principles of economics to healthcare sector.

1.2 Health Care as a Commodity

The focus of economics is on the demand, supply and distribution of commodities. Health has value in use but not value in exchange, implying therefore, that health is non-tradable. However, health care is tradable. The consumption activities of an individual help to produce health, but there is no market in which health itself may be traded directly. While a large number of marketable commodities affect health, health care is consumed specifically and singularly in relationship to health. Health care is only consumed on the presumption that it has investment benefits for health status. The demand for health care is, therefore, a derived demand based upon the consumer's desire for health which in turn is desirable for the full enjoyment of all other production and consumption activities.

1.3 Health Care Services

The purpose of health care services is to improve the public health status through reduction of mortality and morbidity, thereby, increasing the life expectancy. The Alma-Ata Declaration (1978) emerged as a major milestone for public health in the twentieth century. It identified primary health care as the key to the attainment of the goal of "Health for All". The Millennium Development Goals (MDG, 2000) aims to reduce poverty, hunger, ill health and gender inequality. The Millennium Development Goals 5(MDG5), 2005 aims to improve maternal health. Recognizing the importance of health in the process of improving quality of life, thereof, economic and social development the government of India launched National Rural Health Mission on 5th April 2005. The state of Arunachal Pradesh implemented it since 8th September 2005. NRHM includes various components such as Reproductive and Child II, the National Disease Control Programme Revised National TB Control Programme (RNTCP), National Vector Borne Disease Control Programme (NVBDCP), and National Programme for Control of Blindness (NPCB), The National Leprosy Eradication Programme (NLEP), Integrated Disease Surveillance Programme (IDSP), and Iodine Deficiency Disorder Control Programme (IDDCP), integrated disease surveillance project and main streaming AYUSH.

1.4 Maternal Health and Maternal Health Care Services

1.4.1 Meaning

Promoting health behaviours and increasing knowledge on pregnancy and pregnancy related complications among women, families and communities are essential to health and well being of women in general. Maternal health refers to the health of the mother during pregnancy, child birth and post partum period. Maternal health care services include antenatal care, safe delivery and post natal care.

1.4.2 Antenatal care

Antenatal care is the care of the woman during pregnancy. The primary aim of antenatal care is to achieve at the end of a pregnancy a healthy mother and a healthy baby. Ideally this care should begin soon after conception and continue throughout pregnancy. Ideally the mother should attend the antenatal clinic once a month during the first 7 months; twice a month, during the next month; and thereafter, once a week, if everything is normal. A high proportion of mothers in India are from lower socio-economic group and many of them are working women. Attendance at the antenatal clinic may mean loss of daily wages. Consequently, it is difficult for them to attend the antenatal clinic so often. In these case a minimum of three visits covering the entire period of pregnancy should be the target, as shown below:

1st visit at 20 weeks or as soon as the pregnancy is known

2nd visit at 32 weeks

3rd visit at 36 weeks

Further visit may be made if justified by the condition of the mother. At least one visit should be paid in the home of the mother.

1.4.3 Institutional Delivery

These are deliveries that take place in health facilities; public and private hospitals/clinics with maternal care services. About one percent of deliveries tend to be abnormal and four percent "difficult", requiring the services of a doctor. Institutional care is recommended for all "high risk" cases, and where home conditions are unsuitable. The mother is allowed to rest in bed on the first day after delivery. From the next day, she is allowed to be up and about. The current practice is to discharge the woman after 5 days lying-in-period after a normal delivery.

Health institutions should be well equipped with well trained and motivated staff, with adequate drug supply and equipments and be able to provide effective emergency obstetric care within an enabling environment. While any woman can develop complications at any stage of pregnancy; most if not all such complications can be managed effectively. Interventions that are benefits to mothers help babies too. Thus, utilising health facilities for delivery is critical for the live of the pregnant woman and that of her unborn child.

1.4.4 Postnatal Care

Care of the mother after delivery is known as postnatal and is extended upto the first six weeks after birth. This period is critical to the health and survival of a mother and her newborn. The most vulnerable time for both is during the hours and days after birth. Lack of care in this time period may result in death or disability as well as missed opportunities to promote healthy behaviours, affecting women, newborns, and children. Yet the postnatal period receives less attention from health care providers than pregnancy and childbirth.

In order to improve maternal health, the Government of India has initiated various programmes such as the National Rural Health Mission (2005-2012) which was launched by the Government of India (GoI) in 2005 to provide effective health care to rural population in the country with special focus on states with poor health outcomes and inadequate public health infrastructure including manpower. Its primary focus is to improve access to health care services by rural people, especially women and children in an equitable and affordable way. As such, one of primary goal of NRHM is to reduce Infant Mortality Rate (IMR) and Maternal Mortality Ratio (MMR) by promoting newborn care, immunization, antenatal care, institutional delivery and post-partum care.

The Reproductive and Child Health Programme was launched throughout the country on 15th October, 1997. Later on, in 2005, RCH II was merged with NRHM to cater to accessible maternal health care in the rural areas. The programme aims at achieving regulated fertility, safe antenatal, post natal as well as safe child birth. Reproductive Health is not merely the absence of disease or disorder of the reproductive processes, but is a condition in which reproductive functions and processes can be accomplished in a state of physical, mental and social well being. It is envisaged to provide an integrated package of services. First, it includes services for mothers during pregnancy, child birth and post-natal period. It also includes service to newborn like immunisation which includes from vaccination to giving of Vitamins, Oral Rehydration Therapy (ORT) and management of Acute Respiratory Infections (ARI). Further it also includes contraception, preventative and counselling services.

With regard to the objective of reducing maternal and neonatal mortality by promoting institutional delivery among pregnant women, the JSY was incorporated in NRHM. The scheme encourages pregnant women to undergo at least four antenatal check-ups and go for institutional delivery rather than at home by providing cash assistance. The scheme is emphasised in states where institutional delivery rates are low. Under the scheme institutional deliveries either in government or accredited private health facility are entitled to Rs 1400 in rural areas and Rs 1000 in urban areas in low performing states. In high performing states, pregnant women are entitled a sum of Rs 700 in rural areas and Rs 600 in urban areas. Government of India also launched Janani Shishu Suraksha Karyakaram since 1st June, 2011. It entitles all women to deliver child, including caesarean section absolutely free. Further it entitles free services like drugs and consumables, essential diagnostics, diet during stay in the health institution, provision of blood and pick and drop facility.

1.5 Global and National Scenario of Maternal Health

The status of health care services is one of the critical measures particularly mother's health. Maternal health is mother's health during pregnancy, childbirth and in post natal period. Maternal health is important to communities, families and the nation due to its profound effects on the health of the women, immediate survival of the newborn and long term well being of children, and well being of families. Maternal death and illness have cost implications on family and the community because of high direct and indirect costs, the adverse impact on productivity and the human tragedy that every maternal or child death represents due to maternal or infant death can be reduced. Therefore, investigations are essential in this period by timely diagnosis of complications and likely problems which women can face during the process of child birth. This can be provided if the women have access to maternal health care services. Globally, an estimated 2,87,000 maternal deaths occurred in 2010 of which 99 percent were in the developing countries. Only half of the women in developing regions received the recommended amount of health care needed[1]. In India, around 78,050 pregnant women die every year during pregnancy i.e. for every one lakh live births, 301 maternal deaths occurs on the average[2].Maternal death in India accounts for nearly 19 (56 000) of the global total.

The global MMR in 2010 was 210 per 100 000 live birth. In contrast to global rank of 9th place for political empowerment, it has ranked second-lowest position for health and survival out of 136 countries (World Economic Forum, 2013). Although the Maternal Mortality Rate (MMR) in India dropped from 212 per 100000 live births in 2007-2009 to 178 in 2011-12, it is still high. Only one out of every 24 infant in the national level, 22 infant in rural and 36 infants in urban areas survives[3]. As mothers who expires during first 6 weeks makes the infant more prone to termination in the first two years of life, the MMR has a direct impact on infant mortality rate (IMR). The Infant Mortality Rate (IMR) in India is 44 per 1000 live birth in the first year of a child's life (SRS, 2012). During 2013, India ranked as low as 136th position among 186 countries. As for maternal healthcare services, only 44 per cent of women started antenatal care in the first trimester of pregnancy. The Human Development Report, 2011, listed North Eastern states under Medium Human Development Index (0.573) except Assam. It further rates MMR below national average except Assam and Meghalaya[4].

1. WHO, UNICEF, UNFPA and The World Bank estimates, Trends in mortality 1990-2010
2. Sample Registration Survey - 2001-02
3. Register General Of India, 2013 [7] SRS 2007-2009
4. Global Health Observatory, www.who.int/gho

The health scenario of Arunachal Pradesh stands comparatively much behind the rest of India. The most recent data available on maternal mortality rate in Arunachal Pradesh was 337 per 100000 live births (SRS, 2005). The HDI ranking was 15th among the 28 states in case of Arunachal Pradesh. The IMR for the state is 32 per 1000 live birth. Government of India has been continuously putting effort in attempt to improve the maternal health, especially in rural areas through National Rural Health Mission. This is reflected in the various schemes like JSY and JSSK which have attracted the rural women to access maternal health care services. Since many of the health problems during pregnancy can be prevented, detected and treated, a minimum of four antenatal visits, comprising interventions such as vaccinations, screening and treatment for infections and identification of warning signs are usually prescribed for. It is this reason that maternal health care services become eminent. World over, during 2005-2012, about 55 of pregnant women attended the recommended minimum antenatal care, while the rest of 45 are not fortunate to access such health care due to various reasons. Though dismal, access to maternal/antenatal care has increased from 37 in 1990 to about 50 in 2011 for high income nations whereas it is 37 for low income countries. In case of India, it was reported to be 75.20 in 2008[8]. National Family Health Survey-3 (2005-2006) revealed that only 44 per cent of Indian women started antenatal care in the first trimester of pregnancy. The percentage of women getting more than three antenatal visits by the Auxiliary Nurse Midwife (ANM) ranged from 17 per cent in Bihar and Uttar Pradesh to 90 per cent in Kerala, Goa and Tamil Nadu. The percentage of women who received two or more tetanus toxoid vaccination ranged from 40 per cent in these States to 90 per cent or more in areas like Delhi, West Bengal and Tamil Nadu. About 16.3 percent of mother receives full ANC which includes at least three ANC checkups, one TT injection and 100 Iron Folic Acid tablet/ syrup consumed. Although the percentage of mother receiving full ANC is low, on the average about 69.8 percent receives at least once ANC. Further, about 70 percent of women opt for institutional deliveries but the proportion of newborn check-up within 24 hours after birth is as low as 39.9 percent and 60.1 percent have no check-ups within 10 days after birth. However, the Health Management Information System (HMIS, 2013-14) showed that the institutional delivery in the state is 33.8 percent while for the mother with three or more ANC is 39.67 percent which is very low. The utilisation of these services differs spatially from district to district and from urban to rural areas. The study is therefore an attempt to highlight the status and the factors that determines the use of MHC services in rural areas as well as its barriers.

Chapter - II

Literature Review

High rate of maternal mortality in developing countries has become a matter of great concern for the world today. Therefore, improving maternal and child health are two basic objectives of the Millennium development goals. The goal specified in Millennium Development Goal-5 (MDG 5) is to reduce the maternal mortality ratio by 75 by 2015. India is one amongst the countries where MMR is high. There are about 212 maternal deaths per 100,000 live births which translate into about 56,000 pregnant women or new mothers dying annually, often from preventable causes (Priyanka Dixit, 2013). The country's MDG target is to reduce the maternal death to 109 per 100,000 live births by 2015.

Majority of these deaths takes place in rural areas where maternal health care is poor. Studies reflect that in India over 95, of maternal deaths occur among women who have never received ANC. In spite of all efforts by the government, only 12 of women in the rural areas receive ANC. The leading causes of this grim outcome are infections, haemorrhage, anaemia and pre-eclampsia which can be prevented through better access to health services (Dr.Huma Rathore). Hence, provision for better ANC is critical, especially in the rural areas of developing countries to anticipate complications which if taken care, can further improve maternal health (Alehagen et al, 2012).

A study in rural India (Aligarh) found that majority of women did not have ANC check-up. Amongst those women who had ANC check-ups, women who had three or more ANC checkups were insignificant (Ansari and Khan, 2011). It is believed that increased awareness of preventive health care and education lead to patient-friendly encounter between health professionals and patients which might decrease maternal and child mortality (Alehagen et al, 2012). Nevertheless, ANC itself is inadequate in preventing maternal and child deaths, unless supported by institutional delivery and post natal care.

The Article 25 of Universal Declaration for Human Rights (1948) recognised motherhood and childhood as entitlement and urges for special care and assistance. The vision of the World Health Organisation (WHO) in 'Making Pregnancy Safer' advocates for skilled care for all during pregnancy, childbirth and immediate post natal period. While approximately half of the world's women have skilled birth attendant present during delivery, the proportion is highly skewed. Three quarters of urban women have an attended birth and only about one-third of rural women have skilled attendant during delivery. Achieving 80 per cent institutional deliveries and conducting 100 per cent deliveries by trained personnel had been considered crucial in the National Socio-Demographic Goals 2010, of Government of India. But a study suggests that majority of the births particularly in the rural areas, are still delivered at home (Garg et.al, 2010). Considering this, the government of India has assigned the primary role to Accredited Social Health Activists (ASHAs) under National Rural Health Mission (NRHM) to bring the pregnant mothers to government hospitals for delivery purpose. However, it has not been successful to attract the beneficiaries to the expected level. Even offering cash incentives under Janani Suraksha Yojana (JSY) for getting ante-natal care (ANC) and for institutional deliveries, the attraction is below expected level (Roy et.al, 2013).

The response to JSY is however uneven. Qualitative study in rural Uttar Pradesh found that the introduction of JSY accelerated the adoption of institutional delivery (Varmal et.al, 2010). This is supported by another study in Karnataka, where it was found that the implementation of JSY has increased the number of institutional deliveries and reduced infant mortality rate significantly (Mamatha and Navitha, 2014).

With the advancement in technology, child birth has come under the influence of medical technology through medicalisation of human body both theoretically and empirically in the past decades. Medicalisation is a process by which health or behaviour problems come to be defined and treated as medical issues. One example of the medicalisation of the human body is caesarean-section (c-section) delivery. With the increase in institutional deliveries and growing access to gynaecological and obstetric care, c-section deliveries too have shown an increasing trend in India (Sancheetha Ghosh, 2010). As women's health is critical even after delivery as it affects the child's health, postnatal care is a necessity. It influences the health of both the mother and child greatly. Postnatal care is most common following births in a medical facility; however, about one in five births in medical facilities do not follow up postnatal check-ups. The WHO recommended the first postnatal contact as early as possible within 24 hours of birth at home. However, only 15 percent of home births followed postnatal check-ups (NFHS-3, 2005-06). Thus, not only non-institutional deliveries but no post partum care is also predominant in rural areas. Traditional postpartum practices are prevalent among women in rural Malaysia where self-belief forms the basis for the practices of traditional postpartum care (Hishamshahz et al, 2013). Similarly much of women behaviour during postnatal period was strongly influenced by cultural background (Mangalore), India (Sunanda B and Shynee Paul, 2013). During the first Week after delivery at home or institutions, women suffered a high burden of morbidities and severe anaemia. The study suggested that Health programmes should invest to ensure that all women receive early postpartum visits after delivery at home or after being discharged from institutions to detect and manage maternal morbidity. In fact, health programmes should also ensure that women are properly screened for complications before their discharge from hospitals after delivery (Kirti Iyengar, 2012).

2.1 Factors Associated with the Utilisation of Maternal Health Care Services

Studies suggest that utilisation of maternal health care services are determined by a number of factors. The desire to be pregnant or become mother also has often captured in the determination of maternal health care utilisation (Erlindawati et al; 2008). Unintended pregnancy is an important public health problem that predisposes women to maternal deaths, through unsafe abortions and poor maternity care (Wado et al; 2013).

Self motivation and knowledge about health care services seeks to increased utilisation of it. Motivations from husband, relatives or health professionals are also a determinant to the access of maternal health care services. Nevertheless, husband education was found to be having stronger impact on the utilisation of maternal health care services (Chakroboty et al, 2003). Therefore, improving the status of women by expanding educational opportunities, strengthening promotion of antenatal and delivery care (DC) by enhancing community awareness about the importance of ANC and DC are recommended (Birmeta et.al; 2013).

The characteristic of women also occupy an important place in the determination of maternal health care use. Freedom of choice and making decision has been found to be an important dimension of women's autonomy in this setting. Its associations with maternal health care utilisation suggests that even in traditional societies, where women had limited autonomy, freedom pertaining to women's mobility can have an important bearing upon their health behaviour (Bloom et al, 2001).

Family structure and organisation also enters into determination of maternal health care. In this regard the family structure implies either joint or nuclear family. Often, women belonging to nuclear family have been found to use antenatal care more than those in the joint family in urban areas and had better knowledge about antenatal care in India (Lausharam et al; 2013). Contrarily, women in joint families get more maternal health care due to family support that is not available in nuclear households. Thus, women in joint families are in more contact with family members and receive more encouragement to seek care (Conrad et.al; 1998).

The use of maternal health care services was also found to be varying among the scheduled tribe's women from region to region. It was found that tribal women of North-Eastern states were twice as likely to deliver in institution compared to those of central India, 54 percent more likely to receive assistance from trained health professionals for delivery but less likely to receive complete antenatal care services than the women of central states(Shah and Belanger; 2011). In addition, the community factor also shaped the level of use of maternal health care services, such as the presence of anganwadi centre in a village. The effectiveness of the anganwadi, in this respect, provides a rationale for expanding the range of health information and primary care available at the centre for maternal and child health (Sharan, 2005).

In India, the use of maternal health care services varies depending upon religion and caste. Those who belonged to Hindu religion, particularly general caste were more likely to use antenatal care and institutional delivery than others and more than Muslim and scheduled tribe's mothers (manna et al; 2011). However, adequate studies suggested otherwise. In one of such studies, Hindu women were least user while Muslim women received not only more, but all the three dimensions of maternal health care services (Jat et al; 2011). Thus, the argument was reduced to relative non-utilisation of maternal health care by tribal study. Women who followed traditional belief system were less likely to use maternal health services than any other groups (Mekonnen and Mekonnen, 2002).

Poor attitude of health care workers especially in public hospitals, have deterred many women from utilising maternal health care services. It was generally felt that the absence of a suitable waiting shelter designed for expecting mothers was contributing factor to the low use of institutional delivery services (J. Stekelenburg et al; 2004).

The place of residence also influences the use of maternal health care. High level of utilisation of maternal health services among urban women were found compared to their rural counterpart, as health facilities are more accessible in urban areas. Further, rural women were found to be more readily influenced by traditional practices, contrary to modern health care (Mekonnen and Mekonnen, 2002).

In India, the inter-regional diversity is an important factor determining the use of maternal health care. Amongst the different components of maternal health care services, use of antenatal care varied from 32 in Rajasthan to 98 in Kerala. The coverage for vaccination (tetanus) was more than 90 in Kerala, Tamil Nadu, and Goa, while it was 45 in Uttar Pradesh, Madhya Pradesh, and Rajasthan. Less than 30 of mothers in Nagaland, Bihar, and Uttar Pradesh received iron and folic acid tablets, while it exceeded 84 in Kerala, Goa, and Tamil Nadu. The percentage of institutional delivery was 88 in Kerala, and Goa, and it ranged from 11 to 12 in Uttar Pradesh, Bihar, and Assam (Gokhale et al; 2002).

Birth preparedness i.e. preparations for childbirth made by pregnant women, their families, and communities increases the use of skilled birth attendants (SBAs) and reduces maternal morbidity and mortality. Birth preparedness, and skilled birth attendant, can be enhanced through mass media (Gustav Asp et. al.; 2013).

Exposure to mass media provides increased awareness and knowledge, as well as changes in attitudes, social norms and behaviours. It leads to positive public health outcomes. Therefore, policy efforts in improving education, spreading health care information through media and providing a better local network of health workers will go a long way in augmenting development through improving the health of the mother and the child (Sheriff and Singh, 2002).

As pregnancy is perceived as a natural process of life, women; families and communities may underestimate the importance of antenatal care. A popularisation is that of going to institution for delivery as futile; acts as a barrier to access of the maternal health care. As such, the use of these services is also influenced by the factors like ignorance of antenatal care facilities (Birmeta et al; 2013). Therefore, perception regarding antenatal care as well as awareness contributes a lot to the utilisation of maternal health care. In addition to it there should also be the willingness and the ability to access such services.

Hence, both awareness of the need for institutional delivery and the ability to go to a medical institutions are important determinants to the access of maternal health care (Digamber et.al; 2011).

It is also perceived that better educated women are more aware of health care services and use the information more effectively to maintain or achieve good health status. Thus, with the increased in the level of education, the adequacy of knowledge, thereof awareness, also increases and so thus use of ANC. As such, Mother's education was found to be the most important factor that determines the use of maternal health care services (Matsumina and Gubhaju; 2001). Studies also suggested that most of the women were aware of maternal health care services, in general, but lacked the comprehensive knowledge. So with higher level of education, the utilisation of the maternal health services increased (Olayink et al; 2013). A similar result was concluded in a study where mother's education positively impacts the maternal health care utilisation (Govindasamy and Ramesh; 1997). Moreover women with primary education and secondary education were found utilising antenatal care and health facility for delivery than the illiterate (Assfaw et al; 2010).

Important factor which affects the decision to utilise maternal health care is wealth status of the individuals. The wealthier the family is, more likely it is for a women to access ANC and deliver her baby with professional birth attendance (Desai et al; 2006). As such, lower the income and wealth strata of the family, more intense are the rate of non-utilisation of maternal health care services. Women from families living below poverty line are less likely to use maternal health service comparing to women above poverty line (Jat et al; 2008).

A strong correlation between birth order and use of maternal health care services was also suggested by number of studies. There is growing awareness about maternal health care and of maternal healthcare facilities. It is, therefore, expected that an efficient use of such facilities will be realised at greater intensities. Younger women are therefore, more likely to access maternal health care services than the older one (bloom et al; 2001). Nevertheless, contrast to it studies also suggested that middle aged women preferred more the institutional delivery than young ones (Salaam et al; 2006). Generally, it is felt that due to the perceived risk associated with first pregnancy, women are expected to seek maternal health care services in first birth order (Thind et al; 2008). This generally was found contradictory as it was found that maternal health care services were often sought during second order birth, and it decreased with birth order more than two (Jat et al; 2011). Such might be due to the fact that the expectant mothers are already experienced to take care of the subsequent pregnancies. Hence use of these services decrease with increasing birth order (Arthur, 2012).

The health of mother depends partially on their access to maternal healthcare services and is an important determinant in its utilisation, socially in developing countries. Because of the high cost associated with the services, the poor are less likely to access maternal health care services. As time allocation for women in the rural areas for acquiring health facilities are limited due to pre-occupation with the household activities, the distance from the health facilities influence the use of maternal health care services. Inadequate transportation facility especially in remote areas and poor road conditions can make it extremely difficult for women to reach even relatively nearby facilities. Thus, closer the distance to health facility, more was the utilisation of ANC, postnatal care and delivery in health facilities (Sharan et al; 2005). There are numbers of literatures which studied the determinants of utilisation of maternal health care services in different parts of India. But no literatures are available in the context of Arunachal Pradesh; except some reports in the health department.

2.2 Objectives of the Study

Based on the above reviews of available literature the following are the objectives of the study:

1. To study the socio-economic profile of the study area.
2. To examine the status of maternal health care.
3. To identify the barriers to the utilisation of maternal health care.

2.3 Organisation of the Chapters

The study is organised in the following way:

Chapter I comprises of the introductory statement, statement of the problem, the objectives of the study and the area of the study.

Chapter II consists of the brief review of the existing literature on maternal health care services.

Chapter III focuses exclusively on the database and methodology.

Chapter IV enumerates the socio-economic profile of the study area and the socio-economic characteristics of the household surveyed.

Chapter V deals with the analysis of data, results and discussion.

Chapter VI includes major findings and conclusions.

Chapter - III

Methodology

Research is a continuous process and if research does not work systematically on problem, there is less possibility to unearth the final result. Hence a proper methodology is needed to be framed to find out the result of a research problem. This chapter discusses the methodology used in details.

3.1 Area of the study

The area of the study is Mebo sub-division of East Siang district. It is situated in the midst of three district headquarters i.e. about 130 kms north from Yingkiong, the district headquarter of Upper Siang; 20 kms East from Pasighat, the district headquarter of East Siang and 125 kms west from Roing, the district headquarter of Dibang Valley District at an altitude of about 342 m above sea level. The area is well linked by P.W.D. and National Highway (NH-52A). It lies roughly between 270 55' N and 280 25' N latitudes and 950 15' E to 950 35' E longitudes. There are 18 villages under Mebo sub-division spread over an area of 810.746 Sq.km. The name of the villages are Mebo, Ayeng, Bodak, Silluk, Aohali, Motum, Sigar, Ralling, Kiyit, Ngopok, Borguli, Seram, Kongkul, Namsing, Mer, and Gadum. Further it is divided into two blocks i.e. Mebo- Banggo and Monggu Banggo. The first eight villages come under Mebo-banggo and the rest six villages come under Monggu-Banggo. It has a total population of 14474 out of which 7381 are males and 7093 are females (Census, 2011). The area is inhabited by Adi, Idu Mishmi and Mishing Tribes. Agriculture is the main occupation. There is one community health centre (CHC), two primary health centres (PHCs) and four sub-centre (SCs) in the study area.

3.2 Design of the Study

The study is descriptive in nature and cross-sectional in design. Cross-sectional studies provide a "snapshot" of the outcome and the characteristics associated with it at a specific point of time. Thus, it has the advantage of avoiding various complicated aspects in the use of data drawn from various points of time. Considering previous studies and knowledge it was considered indispensable to use both qualitative and quantitative methods. By using both qualitative and quantitative tools, more rigorous and rich data can be collected and this is expected to enrich and improve the findings of the study.

3.2.1 Quantitative Methods

The quantitative part reviews the socio-economic profile of the surveyed villages. It also includes the characteristics of the women who had at least one delivery during the last five years preceding the survey. Data was collected using structured questionnaire in which both open and closed ended question were included. Characteristics of women was collected to determine past pregnancies, age of the women during last birth, level of education, number of antenatal visit, persons who advised women to go maternal health care and occupation of the women.

3.2.2 Qualitative Methods

This part of the study was done to explore, in depth, the contributing factors to a broader picture from women's experiences and knowledge. The main aim was to engage women to tell their own reasons for non-utilisation of maternal health care services.

3.3 Sampling and Tools

This section includes the sampling and tools used in the study. Under this the following sub-heading has been worked out:

3.3.1 Sample Size and Selection

For quantitative part, sample size was determined by the number of households in a particular village. From each selected villages 15 percent of the household were covered. The attempt was made to select more villages of the study area to make the sample more representative. Out of 18 villages, 14 villages were covered in the field survey. The total number of household surveyed was 279. As the sampling was purposive in nature only those households in which women had at least one delivery in the last five years preceding the survey, were selected for interview. The purposiveness of sampling was further disaggregated to snow balling techniques. Snowballing is a purposive sampling approach, where one participant gives the researcher the name of another subject, who in turn provides the name of another, and so on. It works as a chain sequence of recommendation or introduction from one respondent to another. Snowballing offers many practical advantages as it helps the researcher to identify people of interest from other people the researcher has interacted with. In this way the women qualifying for interview in the village or in other villages were identified. The villages that could not be covered are likely to have same characteristics of the nearest villages that were covered. As the study includes only those women who had at least one delivery during the last five years preceding the survey, only 15 percent of the total household in bigger villages were interviewed. In case of small villages like Aohali and Bodak all of them were interviewed. Those women who have no particular response were included in "not responded properly" category.

3.3.2 Statistical Tools

For the quantitative part, a structured questionnaire was used to collect the required information relating to mother's age, level of education, mother's occupation, past pregnancies and deliveries complications, number of antenatal visit, persons who advised them to go maternal health care was developed. Qualitative method was used to collect information on 'yes' or 'no' answer. They were asked whether they received maternal health care or not, if not why? Both methods were pilot tested.

The data obtained from primary sources have been analysed using descriptive statistics for both socio-economic profile and status of utilisation of maternal health care as well as barriers to these services. Cross tabulation of the data was made in order to associate the various factors like educational level of mother, age, occupation etc. with utilisation of maternal health care services.

3.4 Selection of Variables

Variables were selected keeping in mind the objectives of the study. The socio and economic conditions of sample respondents are studied by analyzing the respondent's position with respect to literacy level, occupation, land holdings, family size etc. which are explained below. The determining factors associated with the utilisation of maternal health care services have been taken from the review of existing literature.

3.4.1 Socio-Economic Variables

The socio-economic variables were calculated based on the total population of the sample households. It was measured by taking different variables as follows:

1. Level of education: Education can improve the human capital of an individual and the human resources of a nation. The increase in the level of education particularly of women will reshape the untapped developmental resource of the family. Hence it is likely to enhance the status of the family. The level of education was categorise into six: no schooling (0 year of schooling), primary (1-5 years of schooling), middle (6-8 years of schooling), secondary (9-10 years of schooling), higher secondary (11-12 years) and degree and above (13+ years of schooling). Those who have attained the age of 5 years and above but never attended school were included in "no schooling" category.

2. Occupational status: The economic status of the people depends on their income generating occupation. As such the occupation of the household was examined. It was divided into four categories. Student category was also included in addition to farmers, services and other categories. Others category includes politicians, business man, wage labour, unemployed or any activities that does not come under farmers, services and students categories. Students are those who are studying. They are included in separate category bearing in mind that they represent a number of populations.

3. Land holdings: The land holding indicates the status of an individual household. The land holdings of the household head are divided into six categories: Marginal (less than 1 hectare), small (1-1.99 hectares), semi-medium (2-3.99 hectares), medium (4-9.99 hectares), large (10 and above hectares) and no land holding. The "no holding" is included because few respondents were labour and tenant who does not hold land.

4. Crops grown and produced: Agriculture is the main occupation of the people in the study area. Therefore, data is also capture to know the type of crops grown and produced by them which helps them in the income generation.

5. Family size: In order to know the size of the family, all the members living in the family were noted down. Under this not only the children of household were included but also the kith and kin that were living with them. It was further divided into three categories: family with 3-5 members, 6-8 members and more than 8 members.

6. Composition of population: Age is a key determinant to utilise the potentialities. Age and socio-economic activities are inter-related. The age composition was classified on the basis of classification of age by the Census of India. These includes 0-4 years, 5-9 years, 10-14 years, 15-19 years, 20-24 years, 25-44 years, 45-64 years, 65-79 years and 80+ years.

7. Marital status: Marriage represents a social contract that bonds individuals together in an intimate relationship that can be stress-buffering and socially integrative. Marital status affects access to sources of income and, therefore, economic security and well-being. It was categorised into "currently married", "not married" and "others". Those girls (18 years) and boys (21 years) who have attained the legal age of marriage but not currently married were included in "Not married" category while "others" category include those who are separated, divorced and widow/widower.

8. Religion: Subject was asked about their religion and it was classified into four: Donyi-polo, Christian, Hindu and Muslim.

9. Livestock owned and reared: Since livestock remains as a source of earning, it is included in the socio-economic variable. Question was asked on different types of livestock owned and reared by the villagers.

3.4.2 Mother's characteristics

Since the study is mainly connected to women, women's characteristics were separately analysed. The selected variables for women's characteristics are level of education, age at last birth, occupational status, and birth order, past pregnancy and delivery complication.

3.4.3 Variables taken as Determinants of Maternal Health Care Services

Maternal health care includes Antenatal care, safe delivery and postnatal care. In this study two components of MHC were considered i.e. antenatal care and institutional delivery. Based on the literature review the following variables were taken as the determinants of the maternal health care for this study.

1. Mother's level of education: With the increase in education, knowledge about health care services is likely to increase. As such, mother's level of education was selected as a variable to associate it with the MHC. It was categorised into six groups. They are No education, primary level of education, middle level of education, secondary level of education, higher secondary level of education and degree and above. Those who have never attended school were included in No education category. Those who have attained upto minimum of 1st year and maximum of 5th years of schooling were included in primary level of education and those with 6th years to 8th years of schooling in middle level of education. Further, those who have achieved upto 9-10 years of schooling were included in secondary level of education while those with 11-12 years of education in higher secondary and lastly 13-17 years of schooling was included in degree and above category.

2. Mother's age at last birth: Age of the mother was divided into three groups: 15-19 years, 20-29 years, 30-39 years and 40 and above. This category was made on the basis of division of age group of mother in NFHS.

3. Occupational status of the mother: Mother's occupation was also taken as a variable. It is divided it into four categories: farmers, services, students and others. "Schooling mother" category was also included considering the fact that significant number of population is represented by them. They include the mother who is still studying after child birth. "Others" category includes house wife, politicians, business, wage labour or any activities apart from farmer, services and students.

4. Birth order of the mother: Birth order represents the number of deliveries of the mothers. This was divided into three categories, 1st birth order, 2nd -3rd birth order and more than 3rd birth order. Those who had first delivery was included in 1st birth order. Similarly more than 2nd or 3rd delivery was included in 2nd-3rd birth order category and so on.

5. Distance from the health facility: Earlier study suggested that distance from health facility also determines the utilisation of maternal health care. Distance from the health facility was divided into two categories: 0-5 kms and 6-10 kms from the nearest health facility.

6. Mothers who suffered from any health problems during pregnancy: In this category question were asked on yes or no response. Those mothers who had suffered from any health problems were included in "yes" category and those with no complicacies were included in "no" category. Further any health problems include any diseases which are not necessarily related to pregnancy.

7. Mothers who experience delivery complications during last delivery: Women who had faced delivery complications in previous delivery may have a higher tendency to seek antenatal and delivery care. In this category also question were asked on yes or no response. Those mothers who had experience delivery complications were included in "yes" category and those with no complications were included in "no" category.

3.5 Nature of Data

The data was obtained from primary and secondary data. Secondary data was collected from the official records and government reports like DLHS and NFHS. DLHS is District Level Household Survey collected by the International Institute of Population Science (IIPS), Mumbai with the main objective to provide reproductive and child health database at district level in India for the enhancement of the activities under National Rural Health Mission (NRHM). NFHS is National Family Health Survey conducted under the stewardship of Ministry of Health and Family Welfare with IIPS, Mumbai as the nodal agency mainly to obtain information on population, health, and nutrition in India and each of its 29 states.

For collection of primary data the individual in-depth interview approach was used. This was done to identify the socio-economic profile of the household, factors associated with the utilisation of maternal health care and the reasons for non utilisation of these services. For socio-economic profile head of the household were interviewed. Data was collected using structured questionnaire. The characteristics like age of the mother at last birth, child birth order, level of education, past pregnancies and occupational status of the women were asked. In addition to it number of ANC visit, distance from the health facility and persons who supported or advise her to received maternal health care were also enquired.

3.6 Limitations, Reliability and Validity of the Data

To improve the reliability of data both approaches; quantitative and qualitative response were utilised. In addition structured questionnaire were not limited to closed ended but also included open ended question. The sample size was representative as it covers the 15 percent of the total households of the study area taken from 14 out of 18 villages.

On the other hand, if we see only the delivery case then it represents about 41 percent of the total delivery. According to the official record of Child development project officer office, Mebo, the number of deliveries from January 2009 to June 2014 was 684. Out of which 279 women were interviewed. Thus, it represents about 41 percent of the total women who had at least one delivery during last five years preceding the survey.

3.7 Map of the Study Area

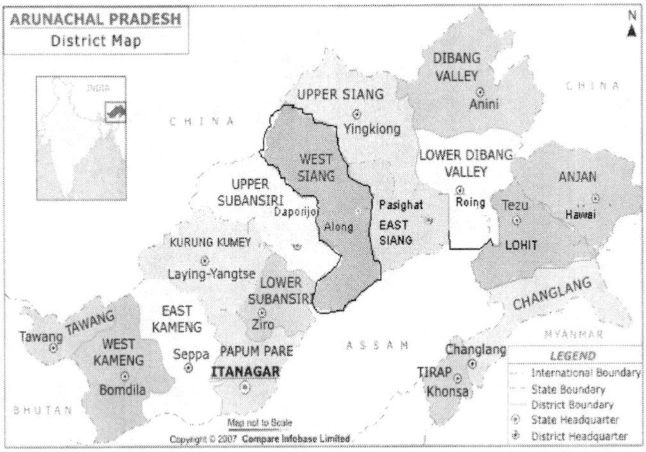

Source: www.imd.gov.in/section/nhac/distforecast/aruanchal pradesh-htm

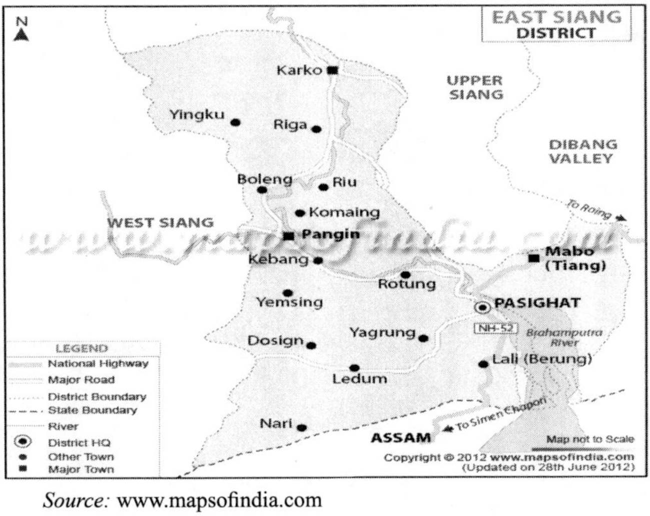

Source: www.mapsofindia.com

Chapter - IV

Socio-Economic Profile of the Study Area

This chapter analyses the socio-economic profile of the study area, which was collected from the primary data. For the socio-economic profile a questionnaire was designed to obtain information. The socio-economic characteristics like, educational status, occupation, age distribution, family size, land holdings, etc. of the sample households have been examined. However, before dealing with the profile of the study area, an attempt has been made to highlight the health profile of the state.

4.1 Profile of Arunachal Pradesh

According to 2011 census, the population of Arunachal Pradesh is 13, 82,611 lakhs. The density of population is 17 persons per square kilometre. If we look at the sex ratio it is below the national average with 920 per 1000 males.

4.1.1 Health Facility in Arunachal Pradesh

There are 3 functional general hospitals including Ramakrishna Mission Hospital in Arunachal Pradesh. The total number of district hospitals is 13 out of which only 12 are functional and that of community health centres is 54, of which only 49 are functional.

Table 4.1: Total number of Health facility in Arunachal Pradesh (Till March 2014)

Facilities	Numbers	Functional
General hospital	3 including RKMH	3
Mental hospital	1	1
District hospital	13	12
Community health centre	54	49
Primary health centre	129	97
Sub-centre	472	286

Source: Official records, NRHM, Naharlagun.

As far as Primary health centre is concerned the total is 129 and the functional is 97. Further, the number of functional sub-centres is 286 but the total is 472. The total number of functional health facilities in Arunachal Pradesh is 448.

4.1.2 Health Human Resources

The effective functioning of the health care depends on the strength of human resources. The existing status of human resources is not adequate to meet up the need of the population. There are only 11 Obstrecian and 7 paediatricians in the state. Based on the IPHS norms the required number of Obstrecian and paediatrician are 76 and 80 respectively. The status of the human resources is shown in Table 4.2. There is a huge shortfall in case of staff nurses (2357) and the existing number is only 233. The total number of existing ANMs is 419 with a shortfall of 365. It is observed that there is a huge shortfall based on the Indian Public Health Standard (IPHS) norms in all the categories of health human resources.

Table 4.2: Health Human Resources in Arunachal Pradesh (Till March 2014)

Discipline	Existing	Shortfall*
Medicine	7	78
Surgery	8	77
Obstrecian	11	76
Paediatrician	7	80
Anaesthesiology	7	78

Ophthalmology	12	58
Orthopaedic	5	11
Pathology	5	13
ENT	3	13
Psychiatric	2	13
Dermatology	1	14
Forensic	1	14
Microbiology	1	14
Epidemiologist	1	16
GDMO(ALLO)	419	334
MO(AYUSH)	67	139
Dental Surgeon	39	31
Staff Nurses	233	2367
Lab Technician	94	167
Radiographer	28	114
Opthal Asstt.	26	44
ECG Tech	5	13
OT TECH	2	247
Pharmacist	201	63
Dental Tech.	21	49
Blood Bank Tech.	0	15
ANM	419	365
HA	319	282

Source: Official records, NRHM, Naharlagun *Based on Indian Public Health Standard norms.

4.1.3 Health Indicators

The percentage of Antenatal care and institutional delivery coverage helps us to know the status of the utilisation of maternal healthcare. Table 4.2 gives us the overview of maternal health care utilisation in Arunachal Pradesh. The percentage of institutional delivery is increasing from 33.7 percent in DLHS-I to 69.9 percent in DHLS-III. Similarly mother who had 3 or more ANC has also increased from 38.4 percent in DLHS-I to 50.4 percent in DLHS-II. However, the recent data based on HMIS shows that institutional delivery and mother who received 3 or more ANC is 38.8 percent and 39.67 percent respectively.

Table 4.3: Status of Maternal Health Care Services in Arunachal Pradesh

Health indicators		DLHS-I (1998-99)	DLHS-II (2002-04)	DLHS-III (2007-08)	DLHS IV (13-14)	HMIS 13-14
Maternal health	Institutional delivery	33.7	47.7	69.9	49.5	38.8
	Mother who had 3 or more ANC	38.4	46.4	50.4	78.3	39.67

Source: Official records, NRHM, Naharlagun, 2014.

4.2. Health facility in Mebo Sub-division

The health services in rural areas are provided through community health centre, primary health centre and sub-centre. There are 1 community health centre, 1 primary health centre and 4 sub-centres in the area. The total numbers of doctors are 12, out of which 6 are Allopathic doctors, 1 child specialist, 1 homeopathy doctors and 1 dentist. The total numbers of nurses are 12. The number of doctors per thousand populations was 0.62 doctors which are below 1 doctor. Similarly the number of nurses per thousand populations was also less than 1 nurse per thousand populations (0.82). The number of beds for indoor patient per one thousand populations was 1.93 beds. This is shown in Table 4.4.

Table 4.4: Numbers of doctors, nurses and hospital beds for indoor patients per 1000 population

Number of doctors/1000 population	0.62
Number of nurses/1000 population	0.82
Number of beds for indoor patient/1000 population	1.93

Source: Own computation, 2014.

4.3 Socio-Economic Profile of the Study Area

As the general trend of the state may or may not apply equally to diverse spatial locations, it is therefore, pertinent to assess the socio-economic profile of the area under study.

4.3.1 Economic Life and Livelihood

Every community has their own way to meet the basic needs for survival. The agriculture is the main economic activity of the people of the study area. It comprises both Jhum and settled cultivation. In addition, hunting, fishing, collection of consumables from forest is the allied usual activity. Jhum cultivation is practiced in the village where source of water for wet rice cultivation is inadequate like Mebo, Silluk, Motum, and Seram.

Settled or wet rice cultivation is mostly practiced where there is adequate source of water like Kiyit, Ngopok and Borguli. Rivers and rivulets remain the main sources of water for irrigation. Few villages like Namsing, Mer and Gadum also practice wet rice cultivation depending on the rain water. The wet rice cultivation for paddy, do not suffice the food habit of the people. As such, they practice to produce chilly, ginger, maize and different kinds of vegetables. The farmers living in Namsing, Mer and Gadum practice crop rotation and dry farming. They grow mustard, potato, cabbage and papad during off agricultural season mainly for marketing purpose.

Domestication of animals is also another important economic activity in this area. Important animals owned and reared are Mithun, cow, pig, goat and poultry. Almost every household domesticate pigs in good numbers. However, the rearing of animals also differs from village to village and from type of livestock in concern. In the lower block, Mithun is generally owned by the few. In few villages like Namsing, Mer and Gadum, Buffalo is considered as an important animal for economic reason while for the upper block Mithun is consider as important animal for social reason. It is sacrificed in solung festival and in some marriage function.

Of late, due to increased connectivity, outlooks as well as economic activities of the people under the study area have undergone rapid changes. With the improvements in the road connectivity to the district headquarter (Pasighat) opportunity of trade and commerce has expanded. Hence in the recent years, along with the usual agricultural products increasing quantities of cash crops like Ginger, orange and sugarcane are being grown in area. In addition to it, vegetables which were earlier grown for consumption purpose are now grown for marketing purposes.

4.3.2 Sources of Income

The level of income determines one's economic status. Since, the majority of the population are farmers the main sources of their income are from agriculture and allied activities including fishing and gathering of forest products. Handlooms and handicrafts also serve as one important source of income for the population concern. Cultivation of commercial crops likes Ginger, mustard and orange contributes a lot to the yearly income of the family. In addition livestock owned and reared also occupy an important place as a source of income. Considering the fact that most of villagers are engaged in agricultural activities and the behaviour of the villagers are more or less likely to be same. No data has been collected for family income assuming that more or less, relatives the level of income as well as the distribution will be same.

4.4 Profile of the Surveyed Villages

In this sub-section, attempt is made to provide a brief account of socio-economic profile of the villages surveyed. In order to obtain data on socio-economic background of the beneficiaries, field surveys were conducted in Mebo-Subdivision in July-August 2014. An attempt was made to cover all the villages under the study area. Out of the eighteen villages, fourteen were covered during field survey. Altogether 279 mothers were interviewed. The total population of the surveyed household is 2054 and the village-wise samples are shown in Table 4.5.

Table 4.5: Name of the Villages Surveyed

Name of villages	*Number of households surveyed*
Mebo	42
Bodak	3
Ayeng	31
Silluk	21
Aohali	5

Motum	19
Ralling	10
Sigar	5
Kiyit	32
Borguli	18
Seram	22
Namsing	44
Mer	18
Gadum	9
Total	**279**

4.4.1 Classification of the Surveyed Household

Education is one of the most important factors contributing to growth and development of the society. It is one of the indicators of quality of human development. The percentage of each level of education of the sample households is shown below in Table 4.4. The given data shows that 28.86 percent had attended primary schooling followed by middle schooling (20.67 percent) and secondary (19.07 percent). It was also seen that 18.33 percent of the total population have no schooling. Only 6.83 percent of the total population had attained "degree and above" education.

Table 4.6: Percentage of Level of Education of the Sample Households

Level of education	*Percentage*
No schooling	18.33
Primary	28.86
Middle	20.67
Secondary	19.07
Higher secondary	6.21
Degree and above	6.83

Source: Own computation from field data, 2014.

4.4.2 Occupational Status of Surveyed Households

Occupational status of the population provides information about the various economic activities that the household is engaged in.

The primary occupation of the surveyed households is shown in Table 5. The field data shows that majority of the population are farmers which accounts for 37.52 percent where as 22.84 percent are school going children. The services and others category contributes 2.88 and 3.42 percents. The people engaged in agricultural are poor which is due to the fact that many growing youths are school dropout. As a result they are compelled to engage in agriculture activities resulting in the highest percentage of farmer among occupational status. Further, the data reveals that school going children are high with 22.84 percent. The analysis of the data brings out that 66.66 percent (sum of farmer, services, in schooling and others) of the total population are engaged in any occupation while 33.34 percent comprises of children, old age and those who are not employed in any activities.

Table 4.7: Occupational Status of the Sample Households

Occupation	*Total number of persons*	*Percentage of total sample population (n=2044)*
Farmers	767	37.52
Services	59	2.88
In schooling	467	22.84
Others	70	3.42

Source: Own computation from field data, 2014.

4.4.3 Classification of Surveyed Households on the Basis of Land Holdings

Agriculture is the main occupation in the surveyed villages. An attempt was made to categorise the households on the basis of size of land holdings. Taking all the sample households together, we find that the average size of the land holdings is around 2.97 hectares. The distribution of size of land holdings are shown in Table 4.8. According to the Table 4.8, the highest percentage falls in the semi-medium category which is 32.3 percent, followed by small category which is 29.2 percent. Only 6.5 percent of the total households have large landholdings. The percentage of marginal and medium landholdings is 8.5 percent and 19.6 percent respectively, while 2.3 percent of the households belonged to landless category.

Table 4.7: Land Holdings of the Sample Households

Category	*Percent*
Marginal	8.6
Small	29.4
Semi-medium	32.3
Medium	19.7
Large	6.5
No land holding	3.6
Total	**100.0**

Source: Own computation from field data, 2014.

4.4.4 Crop production

Different types of crops were found to be grown in study area. The most important as well as significant quantity of output was rice. The list of crops grown and their production in quintals are listed below in Table 4.7. The highest quantity produced is of Rice. In the last year preceding the field survey the amount of rice produced was 6058.50 quintals. This was followed by ginger (1584.80 quintals) and Orange (1040.00 quintals). Mustard, vegetables and others crop were produced with smaller quantities with 342.10, 624.10 and 579.60 quintals respectively. The ginger production is high due to the increasing demand in the market. Although orange production is high, compared to others but its production is confined in a few villages. They are Bodak, Ayeng and countable number of farmer in Mebo villages.

Table 4.8: Crop Production in Last One Year

Crops	Production in quintals
Paddy	6058.50
Ginger	1584.80
Orange	1040.00
Mustard	342.10
Others*	579.60

Source: Own computation from field data, 2014,
* Vegetables, maize, cabbage, potato, papad, etc.

4.4.5 Family Size of the Surveyed Villages (in percentage)

The size of family is crucial in determining the quality of life and the economic status of a household. Attempt was made to identify the population on the basis of family size. Joint family is predominant institution in Aohali village. The size of the family in different categories is more or less same. The size of the family with more than 8 members is 31.5 percent, 31.9 percent for the households with 3-5 family members and 36.6 percent in case of household with 6-8 family members. The overall aggregate average is 7.33 percent.

Table 4.9: Size of the Family of the Sample Household

Family size	*Percentage*
3-5 member	31.9
6-8 members	36.6
more than 8 member	31.5
Average	7.33

Source: Own computation from field data, 2014.

4.4.6 Composition of the Population

The age composition of population is one of the fundamental characteristics of any demographic group. It affects not only demographic but also social, economic and political structure. As such, an attempt is made to examine the age structure of the surveyed villages which are shown below in Table 4.10.

Table 4.10: Composition of Population

Age group		*Percentage of total population(n=2044)*
0-4	419	20.49
5-9	220	10.76
10-14	168	8.21
15-19	161	7.87
20-24	215	10.90
25-44	544	26.61
45-65	282	13.79
65-79	29	1.41
80 and above	6	0.29

Source: Own computation from field data, 2014.

Accordingly, the majority of population are under the age group of 25-44 years (26.58 percent) followed by children between 0-4 years (20.28 percent). The percentage of children (0-14 years) is 39.46 percent while the percentage of working population (15-44 years) is 45.44 percent (highest). The high population in the category of children reveals that the population is increasing. The old age population is very low with only 1.7 percent (65-80+ years) which shows that dependency ratio is less.

4.4.7 Marital Status of the Surveyed Household

As the age structure of the population shows that the highest percentage of population is of the age group 25-44. So the marital status of the population must be relatively high. The marital status of the population is shown below in Table 4.11. It is found that 41.87 percent of the population are currently married, 9.12 percent are not married and 4.42 percent fall in others category i.e. divorce, widow/ widower and separated.

Table 4.11: Marital status of the sample households

Marital status	*Percentage*
Currently married	41.87
Not married	9.12
Others (divorce, widow, separated...)	4.42

Source: Own computation from field data, 2014.

4.4.8 Religion

Religion is one of the indicators that shape the social and cultural identity of the people. The highest concentration of population were found to have faith in Donyi-Polo (68.5 percent) followed by 20.8 percent as Hindu, mostly in the villages bordering Assam. Christian and Muslim constitute 10.0 percent and 0.7 percent of the surveyed population respectively.

Table 4.12: Religion of the sample households

Category	*Percentage*
Donyi-polo	68.5
Christian	10.0
Hindu	20.8
Muslim	0.7
Total	**100.0**

Source: Own computation from field data, 2014.

4.4.9 Livestock Owned and Reared

Tribals are closely associated with the pursuit of domesticating animals. An overview of the types of livestock owned by the villagers is given in Table 4.13. The most commonly owned livestock are pig and poultry. Almost every household, 85.1 percent of the total population practise pigging while 76.2 percent practise poultry. Even though Mithun is considered to be a sacred animal, a very few were found to rear them. Mithun is found to be owned by the villagers of Mebo, Ayeng, Silluk, Bodak, Sigar and Motum. Buffalos are found to be owned by the villagers in the Namsing, Seram and Borguli. The proportion of population who had Mithun and buffalo are 10.3 and 5.3 percent respectively. Further, more than half of the population (52.7 percent) owns Cow.

Table 4.13: Livestock owned and reared by the surveyed households

Name of the livestock	*Percentage*
Cow	52.7
Mithun	10.3
Buffalo	5.3
Pig	85.1
Goat	15.3
Poultry	76.2

Source: Own computation from field data, 2014.

4.5 Conclusion

The socio-economic profile of the surveyed households shows that the percentage of the total sample population who attended schooling is highest in category of primary school (5 years of schooling). Further as the age composition of population are relatively young and children. The marital status is relatively high and hence the population falling under the category of children. The types of crops grown by the villagers are indicative of market orientation, which is encouraging.

Chapter - V

Status of Maternal Health Care Services in Mebo Sub-Division

Any programme of government is successful, if implementation includes the participation of target population or beneficiary. It becomes important to analyse, therefore how the programme is functioning and how the people are responding to it. This chapter focuses on responsiveness of the people to the maternal health care services provided by the health facility. Analysis of the status of utilisation of maternal health care services and the various factors determining the differing use of maternal health care services are carried here in. The barriers that prevent to the access of ANC and institutional delivery have been specially discussed in length.

5.1 Characteristics of Mothers

In this section, village-wise characteristics of mothers are discussed.

5.1.1 Village-wise Percentage of Mothers That Received ANC

Table 5.1 gives us the sample-wise breakup of the ANC received by the target groups

Table 5.1: Village-wise percentage of mothers that received ANC

Name of the village	*No*	*Yes*
Gadum	4 (44.4)	5 (55.6)
Mer	14 (77.8)	5 (22.2)
Namsing	24 (54.5)	20 (45.5)
Seram	3 (13.6)	19 (86.4)
Borguli	1 (5.6)	17 (94.4)
Kiyit	3 (9.4)	29 (90.6)
Motum	10 (52.6)	9 (47.4)
Ralling	1 (20.0)	4 (80.0)
Sigar	1 (10.0)	9 (90.0)
Silluk	3 (14.3)	18 (85.7)
Aohali	1 (20.0)	4 (80.0)
Ayeng	7 (22.6)	24 (77.4)
Bodak	2 (66.7)	1 (33.3)
Mebo	12 (28.6)	30 (71.4)
Total	**86 (30.8)**	193 **69.2)**

Source: Own computation from field survey, 2014.

* Figure within the brackets represents percentage within the village and total represents the overall percentage.

It shows that the respective average ranges from 22.2 percent in Mer which is lowest, to 94.4 percent in Borguli, the highest. In Kiyit and Sigar more than 90 percent of the pregnant women received ANC while sample villages of Seram, Ralling, Aohali, the average ranged in between 80 and 85 percent. It is found that more than 50 percent of the mothers in all villages received ANC, except in Bodak, Motum and Mer. The overall average for all sample villages is 69.2 percent.

5.1.2 Village-wise Percentage of Institutional Delivery

The village-wise percentage of institutional delivery is shown in Table 5.2. The data generated from the field survey reveals that the highest percentage of institutional delivery is observed in case of Ayeng village (64.5). Contrary to it, home delivery is found to be highest in Bodak. In fact, all the deliveries took place at home rather than at health care facility. The sample village with second highest institutional delivery is observed at Aohali (60 percent) followed by Silluk (52.4 percent). Rest of sample villages had on an average institutional delivery less than 35 percent except Kiyit at 46.9 percent. In general, only about 33.3 percent of the mothers had delivered in institution.

Table 5.2: Village wise percentage of Institutional delivery

Name of the village	*Health Facility*	*Home*
Gadum	2 (22.2)	7 (77.8)
Mer	2 (11.1)	16 (88.9)
Namsing	4 (9.1)	40 (90.9)
Seram	7(31.8)	15(68.2)
Borguli	5(27.8)	13 (72.2)
Kiyit	15(46.9)	17(53.1)
Motum	6 (31.6)	13 (68.4)
Ralling	1 (20.0)	4(80.0)
Sigar	5(50.0)	5 (50.0)
Silluk	11 (52.4)	10 (47.6)
Aohali	3(60.0)	2 (40.0)
Ayeng	20 (64.5)	11 (35.5)
Bodak	0 (.0)	3 (100.0)
Mebo	12 (28.6)	30 (71.4)
Total	**93 (33.3)**	**186 (66.7)**

Source: Own computation from field survey, 2014.

*Figure within the brackets represents percentage within the village and total represents the overall percentage.

5.1.3 Mother's Age At Last Birth

Table 5.3 gives us an account of the village-wise percentage of mother in different age group. The highest percentage of mother in the age group of 15-19 years is found in Ralling village (40) followed by Aohali (20), Ayeng (12.9 percent), Mer (11.1 percent), Motum (10.5 percent). No case of mothers in this age group is found in case of sample villages; Seram, Sigar and Bodak. While in rest of the villages such cases were present but are insignificant. The percentage of mother in the age group of 20-29 years is highest in Sigar village (90) and the lowest in Ralling (40 percent) and Aohali (40 percent).

Further, it reveals that more than 50 percent of mothers are of this age group except Aohali (40 percent) and Ralling (40 percent). With the increase in age group from 20-29 years to 30-39 years, the percentage of mothers in the higher age group decreases. The lowest percentage is that of Gadum (11.1 percent) and 40 percent in Aohali is highest. Only in four sample villages the percentage of mothers in this group is more than 30 percent. Those villages include Aohali (40 percent), Silluk (38.1 percent), Bodak (33.3 percent) and Kiyit (31.3 percent).

Table 5.3: Mother's age at last birth

Name of the village	*15-19 years*	*20-29 years*	*30-39 years*	*40 and above*
Gadum	0 (.0)	8 (88.9)	1 (11.1)	0 (.0)
Mer	2(11.1)	10(55.6)	4 (22.2)	2 (11.1)
Namsing	4 (9.1)	35 (79.5)	5 (11.4)	0 (.0)
Seram	0 (.0)	17 (77.3)	5 (22.7)	0(.0)
Borguli	0 (.0)	15(83.3)	3 (16.7)	0 (.0)
Kiyit	2 (6.3)	20 (62.5)	10(31.3)	0(.0)
Motum	2(10.5)	14(73.7)	3(15.8)	0(.0)
Ralling	2(40.0)	2(40.0)	1(20.0)	0(.0)
Sigar	0(.0)	9(90.0)	1(10.0)	0(.0)
Silluk	2(9.5)	11(52.4)	8(38.1)	0(.0)
Aohali	1(20.0)	2(40.0)	2(40.0)	0(.0)
Ayeng	4(12.9)	21(67.7)	5(16.1)	1(3.2)
Bodak	0(.0)	2(66.7)	1(33.3)	0(.0)
Mebo	2(4.8)	30(71.4)	10(23.8)	0(.0)
Total	**21(7.5)**	**196(70.3)**	**59(21.1)**	**3(1.1)**

Source: Own computation from field survey, 2014.

*Figure within the brackets represents percentage within the village and total represents the overall percentage.

As far as the age group of 40-49 years, the percentage of mothers is very less. No mother is found in this age group in all the villages except in Mer (11.1 percent), Ayeng (3.2 percent) and Mebo (1.1 percent). In general, amongst the different age category, the percentage of mothers in the age group 20-29 years is found highest

(70.3) followed by 30-39 years (21.1 percent), 15-19 years (7.5 percent) and 40-49 years (1.1 percent).

5.1.4 Mother's Level of Education

In this sub-section an attempt is made to discuss the mother's level of education in each sample villages. The percentage of each level of mother's education in each villages are given in Table 5.4. It reveals that 21 percent of mothers have never received education, whereas 79 percent of them attended school. In Bodak, it is found that all the mothers had attended schooling. Mothers with no schooling/education is found highest in Mer (66.7 percent) followed by sample village Aohali (60 percent). In case of primary schooling, 17.9 percent of mothers had attended primary schooling. But it varied across sample villages. It is 44.4 percent in Gadum followed by 31.8 percent in Seram, 25 percent in Namsing, 22.2 percent in Mer and Borguli and 15.6 percent in Kiyit. The least is found in Motum (5.3 percent). Amongst the different level of education, the percentage of mothers who attended middle schooling is found highest (32.3 percent). The village-wise comparison shows that it is highest in Silluk (66.6 percent) followed by Ralling (60 percent), Ayeng (48.4 percent), Kiyit (46.9 percent), Motum (36.8 percent), Bodak (33.3 percent) and Ayeng (33.3 percent). The lowest is observed in Gadum (11.1 percent). After achieving the middle schooling, the trend shows that it decreased to 16.5 percent in secondary level. The highest percentage is found in Ayeng (22.6 percent) followed by 22.2 percent in Borguli, 21.9 percent in Kiyit and 20.0 percent in Sigar. It is observed that in every village more than 10 percent of the mother had achieved secondary level of education except in Silluk (9.5 percent) and Motum (5.3 percent). Among all the sample villages, in two villages Bodak and Ralling, none of the mother had achieved this level of education. The highest percentage of mothers who attended higher secondary level of education is observed in Bodak (66.6 percent) followed by Mebo (11.9 percent), Kiyit (6.3 percent) and Borguli (5.6 percent). It is found that none of the mother in Sigar, Aohali, Silluk, Ralling, Mer and Gadum had attended higher secondary level of education.

Table 5.4: Mother's level of education

Name of the villages	*No education*	*Primary*	*Middle*	*Secondary*	*Higher secondary*	*Degree and above*
Gadum	3 (33.3)	4 (44.4)	1 (11.1)	1 (11.1)	0 (.0)	0 (.0)
Mer	12(66.7)	4 (22.2)	0 (.0)	1 (11.1)	0 (.0)	0 (.0)
Namsing	14(31.8)	11(25.0)	8 (18.2)	9 (20.5)	1 (2.3)	1 (2.3)
Seram	4 (18.2)	7 (31.8)	4 (18.2)	4 (18.2)	1 (4.5)	2 (9.1)
Borguli	4 (22.2)	4 (22.2)	3 (16.7)	4 (22.2)	1 (5.6)	2 (11.1)
Kiyit	1 (3.1)	5 (15.6)	15(46.9)	7 (21.9)	2 (6.3)	2 (6.3)
Motum	6 (31.6)	1 (5.3)	7 (36.8)	1 (5.3)	1 (5.3)	3(15.8)
Ralling	2 (40.0)	0 (.0)	3 (60.0)	0 (.0)	0 (.0)	0 (.0)
Sigar	1(10.0)	1 (10.0)	4 (40.0)	2 (20.0)	0 (.0)	2 (20.0)
Silluk	2 (9.5)	3 (14.3)	14(66.7)	2 (9.5)	0(.0)	0 (.0)
Aohali	3 (60.0)	0(.0)	1 (20.0)	1 (20.0)	0(.0)	0 (.0)
Ayeng	2 (6.5)	2 (6.5)	15(48.4)	7 (22.6)	1 (3.2)	4 (12.9)
Bodak	0 (.0)	0(.0)	1 (33.3)	0 (.0)	2 (66.70	0 (.0)
Mebo	5 (11.9)	8 (19.0)	14(33.3)	6 (14.3)	5 (11.9)	4 (9.5)
Total	**59(21.1)**	**50(17.9)**	**90(32.3)**	**46(16.5)**	**14 (5.0)**	**20 (7.2)**

Source: Own computation from field survey, 2014.
*Figure within the brackets represents percentage within the village and of the total represents the overall percentage.

As far as the "degree and above category" is concern, the highest percentage is found in Sigar (20 percent), Motum (15.8 percent) and Borguli (11.1 percent). The least is in Namsing (2.3 percent). It is found that very less percentage of mothers had attained this level of education. In five villages, Gadum, Mer, Ralling, Silluk, Aohali and Bodak, no mother had achieved this level of education. The overall percentage for different categories of education is 21.1 percent in no education, 17.9 percent in primary, 32.3 percent in middle level of education, 16.5 percent in secondary level of education, and 5 percent in secondary level of education and 7.2 percent in degree and above level of education.

5.1.5 Occupational Status of the Mother

The percentage of each category of occupational status of the mother in each sample villages is shown in Table 5.5. The village-wise variation reveals that cent percent of mothers are farmers in Mer, Ralling, Silluk and Aohali. It is found to be lowest in Gadum (55.6 percent). In all the sample villages, it is observed that more than 50 percent of the mothers are farmers. The highest percentage of mothers who is in services is found in Motum (15.8 percent). None of the mother in Gadum, Mer, Namsing, Silluk, Aohali, Bodak and Mebo is found to be in services. Bodak (33.3 percent) recorded the largest number of "schooling mother" followed by Kiyit (21.9 percent), Sigar (10 percent) and Mebo (9.5 percent). No such schooling mother is found in Gadum, Mer, Ralling, Silluk and Aohali. In "others" category Gadum recorded the highest (44.4 percent), Sigar (20.0 percent) and Seram (13.6 percent). Other than these villages it is found insignificant in Namsing (2.3 percent), Ayeng (3.2 percent), Borguli (5.6 percent) and Kiyit (9.4 percent). In general, Data generated from field study shows that the 82.8 percent of the mothers are Farmers. Very few are in services (2.9 percent). It is also found that some of the mothers are still in the schooling as such are put it under "Schooling Mothers" category which constituted 6.8 percent and 7.5 percent in "others" category.

Table 5.5: Occupational Status of the Mother

Name of the village	*Farmer*	*Services*	*Student*	*Others*
Gadum	5 (55.6)	0 (.0)	0 (.0)	4 (44.4)
Mer	18 (100.0)	0 (.0)	0 (.0)	0 (0)
Namsing	42 (95.5)	0 (.0)	1 (2.3)	1 (2.3)
Seram	17 (77.3)	1(4.5)	1 (4.5)	3 (13.6)
Borguli	15 (83.3)	1 (5.6)	1 (5.6)	1 (5.6)
Kiyit	21 (65.6)	1 (3.1)	7 (21.9)	3 (9.4)
Motum	15 (78.9)	3 (15.8)	1 (5.3)	0 (.0)
Ralling	5 (100.0)	0 (.0)	0 (.0)	0 (.0)
Sigar	6 (60.0)	1 (10.0)	1 (10.0)	2 (20.0)
Silluk	21 (100.0)	0 (.0)	0 (.0)	0 (.0)
Aohali	5 (100.0)	0 (.0)	0 (.0)	0 (.0)
Ayeng	27 (87.1)	1 (3.2)	2 (6.5)	1 (3.2)
Bodak	2 (66.7)	0 (.0)	1 (33.3)	0 (.0)
Mebo	32 (76.2)	0 (.0)	4 (9.5)	6 (14.3)
Total	**231 (82.8)**	**8 (2.9)**	**19 (6.8)**	**21 (7.5)**

Source: Own computation from field survey, 2014.

*Figure within the brackets represents percentage within the village and total represents the overall percentage.

5.1.6 Birth Order of the Mothers

Birth order reflects the numbers of deliveries, live or otherwise. The birth order of the mothers is given in Table 5.6. The highest percentage of 1st birth order is found in Seram village (40.9 percent) followed by Aohali (40 percent) and Kiyit (37.5 percent). No mothers of 1st birth order are seen in Ralling village. Most of the mothers had more than one delivery. The three categories of birth order share equal percentage in Mer and Bodak villages with 33.3 percent in each category.

There is a huge variation in more than three birth order from village to village. Whereas all mothers in Ralling (highest) had more than three birth order, it is only about 20.5 percent in Namsing (lowest). It is 40.0 percent in Aohali and Sigar, 33.3 percent in Mer and Bodak and 31.3 percent in Kiyit. More than 20 percent of the mothers in every sample villages had more than three deliveries except Mer (11.1 percent). Out of the total birth order the largest percentage of birth order is concentrated in the "2nd -3rd birth" order (41.9 percent). It is 30.1 percent in 1st birth order and 28.0 percent in birth order more than three.

Table 5. 6: Birth order of the mothers

Name of the village	*1st*	*2nd - 3rd*	*More than three*
Gadum	3 (33.3)	5 (55.6)	1 (11.1)
Mer	6 (33.3)	6 (33.3)	6 (33.3)
Namsing	12 (27.3)	23 (52.3)	9 (20.5)
Seram	9 (40.9)	8 (36.4)	5 (22.7)
Borguli	4 (22.2)	11 (61.1)	3 (16.7)
Kiyit	12 (37.5)	10 (31.3)	10 (31.3)
Motum	6 (31.6)	8 (42.1)	5 (26.3)
Ralling	0(.0)	0(.0)	5 (100.0)
Sigar	1 (10.0)	5 (50.0)	4 (40.0)
Silluk	7 (33.3)	8 (38.1)	6 (28.6)
Aohali	2 (40.0)	1 (20.0)	2 (40.0)
Ayeng	10 (32.3)	12 (38.7)	9 (29.0)
Bodak	1 (33.3)	1 (33.3)	1 (33.3)
Mebo	11 (26.2)	19 (45.2)	12 (28.6)
Total	**117(41.9)**	**78 (28.0)**	

Source: Own computation from field survey, 2014.

*Figure within the brackets represents percentage within the village and total represents the overall percentage.

5.1.7 Village-wise Distance From Nearest Health Facility

Table 5.7 shows the relationship between village-wise distance from nearest health facility and its effect on the ANC and institutional delivery. Nearest health facility includes not only the government Sub-centres, Primary Health Centres and Community Health Centre but also includes health facility run by NGO. The data reveals that out of 14 sample villages, health facility is located within 0-5 kms in 10 villages and 0-6 kms in 4 villages. It is found that more than 50 percent of mothers in all the villages where health facility is located within 0-5 kms access to ANC except Namsing (45.5), Motum (47.4) and Bodak (33.3). The highest is found in Borguli (94.4). However, the percentage of mothers who received ANC where health facility is located more than 5 kms away from their village, it is found very high except in Mer (22.2). The highest is observed in Sigar (90.0), Seram (86.4 percent) and Aohali (80.0 percent).

Table 5.7: Distance from the health facility and its relation with ANC and Institutional delivery

Distance from nearest health facility	*Name of the village*	*ANC Received*		*Place of Delivery*	
		No	*Yes*	*Health Facility*	*Home*
0-5 kms	Gadum	4 (44.4)	5 (55.6)	2 (22.2)	7 (77.8)
	Namsing	24(54.5)	20 (45.5)	4 (9.1)	40(90.9)
	Borguli	1 (5.6)	17 (94.4)	5(27.8)	13(72.2)
	Kiyit	3 (9.4)	29 (90.6)	15(46.9)	17(53.1)
	Motum	10(52.6)	9 (47.4)	6 (31.6)	13(68.4)
	Ralling	1 (20.0)	4 (80.0)	1 (20.0)	4(80.0)
	Silluk	3 (14.3)	18 (85.7)	11 (52.4)	10(47.6)
	Ayeng	7 (22.6)	24 (77.4)	20 (64.5)	11(35.5)
	Bodak	2 (66.7)	1 (33.3)	0 (.0)	3(100.0)
	Mebo	12(28.6)	30 (71.4)	12 (28.6)	30(71.4)
6-10 kms	Mer	14(77.8)	5 (22.2)	2 (11.1)	16(88.9)
	Seram	3 (13.6)	19 (86.4)	7(31.8)	15(68.2)
	Sigar	1 (10.0)	9 (90.0)	5(50.0)	5 (50.0)
	Aohali	1 (20.0)	4 (80.0)	3(60.0)	2 (40.0)
Total		**86(30.8)**	**194(69.2)**	**93 (33.3)**	**186(66.7)**

Source: Own computation from field survey, 2014.

*Figure within the brackets represents percentage within the village and of the total represents the overall percentage.

As far as the institutional delivery is concern, it is highest in Ayeng (64.5) followed by Silluk (52.4) and Kiyit (46.9) which are located within 5 kms from nearest health facility. It is found that there is no institutional delivery in Bodak village. The percentage of institutional delivery is found highest in Aohali (60) which is located beyond 5 kms from the nearest health facility. It is followed by Sigar (50), Seram (31.8) and the lowest in Mer (11.1 percent).

5.1.8 Village-wise Percentage of Mothers Who Suffered From Any Health Problems during Last Pregnancy

A health problem implies any complicacies related to pregnancy and suffering other than it. The percentage of mothers who had any health problems during the pregnancy are shown in Table 5.8. The highest percentage of Mothers who suffered from health problems is found in Ralling (40 percent). Significantly, it is found that no mothers in Motum had suffered from any health problems. More than 30 percent of the mothers had suffered from health problems in Kiyit (37.5 percent), Borguli (33.3 percent) and Mer (33.3 percent). In general, 26.5 percent of the mothers had suffered from health related problems.

Table 5. 8: Village-wise Percentage of Mothers Who Suffered From Any Health Problems

Name of the village	*No*	*Yes*
Gadum	7 (77.8)	2 (22.2)
Mer	12 (66.7)	6 (33.3)
Namsing	33 (75.0)	11 (25.0)
Seram	17 (77.3)	5 (22.7)
Borguli	12 (66.7)	6 (33.3)
Kiyit	20 (62.5)	12 (37.5)
Motum	19 (100.0)	0 (.0)
Ralling	3 (60.0)	2 (40.0)
Sigar	8 (80.0)	2 (20.0)
Silluk	18 (85.7)	3 (14.3)
Aohali	4 (80.0)	1 (20.0)
Ayeng	24 (77.4)	7 (22.6)
Bodak	2 (66.6)	1(33.3)
Mebo	26 (61.9)	16 (38.1)
Total	**205 (73.5)**	**74 (26.5)**

Source: Own computation from field survey, 2014.
*Figure within the brackets represents percentage within the village and total represents the overall percentage.

5.1.9 Village-wise Percentage of Mothers Who Experienced Complications during Last Delivery

In this sub-section, the percentage of mothers who experienced complications during last delivery is discussed.

Table 5.9: Village-wise percentage of mothers who had delivery complications during last pregnancy

Name of the village	*No*	*Yes*
Gadum	8 (88.9)	1 (11.1)
Mer	18 (100.0)	0 (.0)
Namsing	39 (88.6)	5 (11.4)
Seram	16 (72.7)	6 (27.3)
Borguli	12 (66.7)	6 (33.3)
Kiyit	24 (75.0)	8 (25.0)
Motum	18 (94.7)	1 (5.3)
Ralling	4 (80.0)	1 (20.0)
Sigar	6 (60.0)	4(40.0)
Silluk	19 (90.5)	2 (9.5)
Aohali	4 (80.0)	1 (20.0)
Ayeng	23 (74.2)	8 (25.8)
Bodak	3 (100.0)	0(.0)
Mebo	34 (81.0)	8 (19.0)
Total	**228 (81.7)**	**51 (18.3)**

Source: Own computation from field survey, 2014.
*Figure within the brackets represents percentage within the village and total represents the overall percentage.

Table 5.9 shows the village-wise percentage of mothers who experienced complications during last delivery. It shows that the highest percentage of mothers who had complications during delivery is found to be in Sigar (40 percent), Borguli (33.3 percent) and Seram (27.3 percent). It is found that in Mer and Bodak, all mothers did not come across delivery complications. In all sample villages more than 10 percent of the mothers had faced delivery complications except in Motum (5.3 percent). The overall percentage shows that 18.3 of the mothers had delivery complications during last pregnancy whereas 81.7 percent had no complications.

5.2 Status of Utilisation of Maternal Health Care Services

Maternal health care includes antenatal care, safe delivery and postnatal care. Exposure to risk of maternal death increases, if the women do not receive ANC or receives incomplete course of ANC. Maternal health care package for antenatal care (ANC) is one of the major emphasis under NRHM designated under RCH II. ANC comprises of at least three to four physical checks to vaccination and immunisation at periodic intervals during pregnancy to prevent pregnancy related complications. Institutional delivery and post-natal care in a health facility is promoted (NRHM through the Janani Suraksha Yojana) to prevent maternal deaths.

The utilisation of ANC in Arunachal Pradesh is comparatively good. More than fifty percent (50.4) of pregnant women receives ANC irrespective of socio-economic background (DLHS 3, 07-08). The proportion of women who received at least, three ANC is 46.2 percent. About 36.1 percent of women have received first ANC during the first trimester. However, in the recent time, of lately, Health Management Information System (HMIS, 2013-14) reveals that only 39.67 percent of women received three antenatal check-up and the institutional delivery accounts only 38.8 percent.

The utilisation of maternal health care in the Mebo sub-division is far above the state average. About 69.2 percent of women who had at least one delivery in the last five years preceding the survey had received ANC. As far as institutional delivery is concern, it is lower than the state average at 33.3 percent. Further only 17.2 percent of the women and new born received post natal care. The data are shown below in Figure 1. The home delivery (66.7 percent) is found to be twice that of the institutional delivery (33.3 percent). Response to Post natal care is very low as 82.8 percent of the women did not access it. Elaborate attempt on the utilisation of ANC and Institutional Delivery is made in the subsequent sub-section.

Figure 5.1: Maternal Health Care Utilisation in Mebo Sub-Division (percentage)

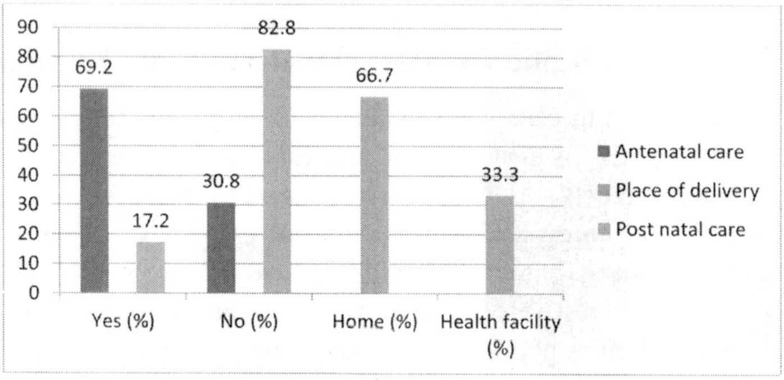

Source: Own computation from field data, 2014.

5.2.1 Utilisation of Antenatal care

In this sub-section attempt is made to analyse about after how many months of pregnancy women went to received ANC for the first time, how many times she received it and who influenced or motivated her to receive ANC. The timing of ANC is important for early detection and diagnosis of any health complications. Figure 5.2 gives us the months of pregnancy at which the mother received ANC. Accordingly, 71.4 percent visited health facility for ANC during the first trimester while 28.6 percent within second-third trimester for the first time. It is also important to know whether the mother received minimum recommended antenatal visit or not. The government through JSY scheme encourages pregnant women to undergo at least four antenatal check-ups. Therefore, mothers who received ANC are classified into three groups with only one time, 2-3 times and 4 and more ANC visits. This is shown below in Figure 5.3. About 50.3 percent of the pregnant women received minimum recommended ANC. Pregnant women who received only one ANC are about 11.9 percent while that of 2-3 times are 37.8 percent.

Figure 5.2: Months at which mother received ANC (in percentage)

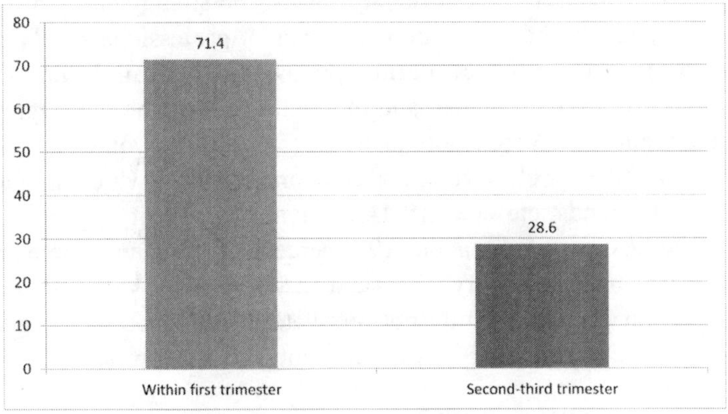

Source: Own computation from field data survey, 2014.

Figure 5.3: Number of ANC visits

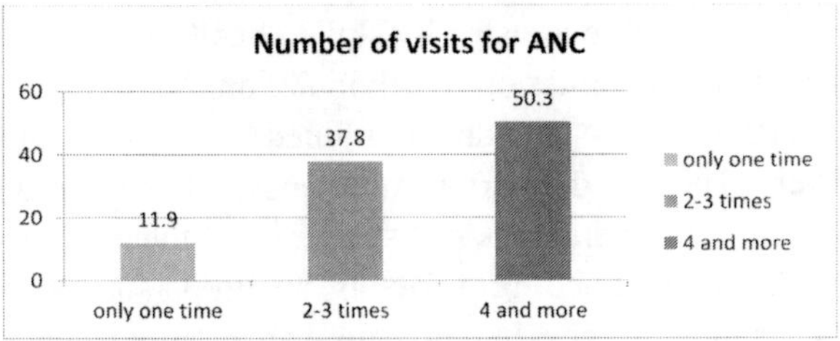

Source: Own computation from field data, 2014.

Figure 5.4: Percentage of women advised for ANC by various categories

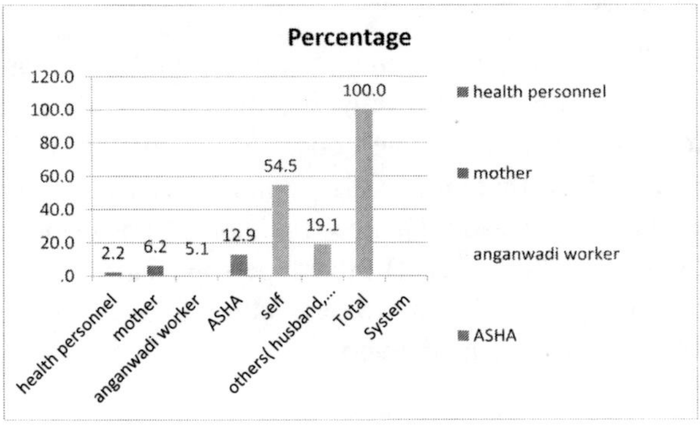

Source: Own computation from field data, 2014.

It is well known that self awareness is important for adoption of health care services. However, it can also be strengthened through encouragement and motivation from health professionals, relatives etc. Therefore, influence during pregnancy to avail health care facilities by encouragement and motivation from others is captured in the Figure 5.4. About more than half (54.5) of the women received ANC based on self awareness category. Others (which includes husband, friends, etc) and ASHA motivated pregnant women to go for ANC. Accordingly, about 19.1 percent of pregnant women are influenced by the category others and 12.9 percent by ASHA workers. The health personnel could not motivate or influence the pregnant women and it accounted only 2.2 percent which is lowest.

5.2.2 Institutional delivery

One of the socio-demographic goals mentioned in the National Population Policy-2000 of India is to achieve 80 institutional deliveries and100 deliveries to be assisted by skilled health personnel by 2015 (India National Commission on Population National Population Policy, 2000). Delivery attended by trained health personnel ensures safe delivery. The first delivery is more unsafe than the others due to psychological reason and lack of experience of the mother. Thus the moral support and advice from friends, health personnel and family members is a must. Hence, in this section an attempt is made to know who conducted the last delivery, who influenced or advice her to deliver in health facility and also whether they received any financial support from JSY or not?

Table 5.10 gives an account of who advised or encourage the mother to go for institutional deliveries. It is found that 31.2 percent of the mothers are aware of the importance of institutional delivery and the reduced risk thereof. It is also found that advice from husband, friends; relatives etc also influenced the mother's decision to deliver in health facility (26.9 percent). Health personnel also contributed as little as 14.0 percent, whereas 15 percent are found to be influenced by mother for institutional delivery.

Table 5.10: Percentage of women advised for institutional delivery by various Categories

Category	Percent
Health Personnel	14.0
Mother*	15.1
Anganwadi Worker	1.1
Asha	11.8
Self	31.2
Others	26.9

Source: Own computation from field data, 2014
*Either mother/ mother-in-law.

The percentage of mother who received financial assistance from JSY is given in Table 5.11. Accordingly only 21.2 percent of the mothers are JSY beneficiaries and the rest of 78.8 percent did not receive any financial assistance. The incentive through JSY is rather over-rated. Contrary to the tall claims, ground realities suggest few members of JSY beneficiaries. Such, instances may be due to uneven distribution of incentives or other non-compliance by the frontline service delivers.

Table 5.11: Percentage of JSY beneficiary

Whether JSY beneficiary?	Percentage
No	78.8
Yes	21.2

Source: Own computation from field data, 2014.

Table 5.12 reveals that about 33.3 percent of deliveries are assisted by health personnel, followed by family members at 28.7 percent. About 22.9 percent of the deliveries are conducted by traditional birth attendant. It is also revealed that 5.7 percent of the deliveries are unattended while 5.4 percent of deliveries are attended by others.

The utilisation of antenatal care is comparatively good as more than fifty percent of the pregnant mother received at least minimum recommended ANC visits of 4. The rest of 49 percent could not receive minimum recommended number of visits. The role played by Health personnel in facilitating mother to receive ANC and of Institutional delivery is very low with 2.2 percent and 14.0 percent respectively. It is found that only 33.3 percent and 3.9 percent of the deliveries are conducted by health personnel and ASHA respectively. More than 20 percent of the deliveries are assisted by traditional birth attendant (22.9 percent) and family members (28.7 percent) whereas 5.7 percent were not attended by any and 5.4 percent were attended by others.

Table 5.12: Persons who assisted last delivery

Category of persons assisting delivery	Percentage
Health personnel	33.3
Traditional birth attendant	22.9
ASHA	3.9
Family members	28.7
None	5.7
Others	5.4

Source: Own computation from field data, 2014.

5.3 Factors Associated with the Use of Maternal Health Care

There are various factors associated with the utilisation of maternal health care. In this section, factors like mother's age, educational level of the mother, birth order etc. are taken in account. The factors associated with ANC and institutional deliveries are also discussed below.

5.3.1 Factors associated with the use of Antenatal care

The various factors that capture the utilisation of ANC are mother's age, mother's education, distance from the health facility, birth order, complications during last pregnancy, mother's occupation, problems during last delivery. The various factors are sub-divided into different categories as shown in Table 5.14.

It is found that the utilisation of ANC decreased with the increase in age, particularly after 29 years. The percentage of utilisation of ANC in the age group 15-19 years is 61.9 percent while in the age group 20-29, it is highest. Thereafter it declined proportionately to 66.1 percent and 33.3 percent for the age group 30-39 and 40 and above respectively.

As far as the level of education is concern, it is found that the percentage of women utilising ANC increases with the increase in education though it is not constant at all levels. 52.5 percent of women with no education availed ANC visits. About 72.2 percent of those who attained primary level education availed ANC while about 74.4 percent of who availed ANC is those who attained middle school level of education. The percentage of those who attained secondary level education is marginally less (65.2 percent). However, it increased to 78.6 percent for those with higher secondary and 90 percent for those with degree and above. In general, with exception to those in the educational category of secondary level, availing of ANC has positive relation to level of educational attainment.

Distance from the health facility is likely to effect the utilisation of ANC. The relationship between utilisation of ANC and distance from the nearest health facility reveals that about 70.1 percent of mother living near health facility avails ANC compared to those living farther (65.5 percent). The utilisation of ANC therefore, decreases with the increase in distance from the health facility. Thus, an inverse relationship between the utilisation of ANC and distance from health facility can be observed.

Utilisation of ANC is also found to be influenced by child birth order. With the increase in the number of births, mother visits for ANC check-up is found to be less. The utilisation of ANC is highest for the first birth order (81.0 percent) followed by 2nd-3rd birth order with 68.4 percent and 57.7 percent in the birth order of more than three. Thus, an inverse relationship is found between the birth order and the utilisation of ANC.

Economic factors are also likely to effect the utilisation of ANC. However, in this study only one aspect of economic status of the occupation of mother is taken into account. Attempt is made to identify the relationship between occupational status of the mother and the utilisation of ANC. The data generated from the field survey reveals that utilisation of ANC increased with higher occupational status of the mother. The percentage of utilisation of ANC by the farmers is 67.5 percent and is 100 percent amongst the mother who are in services. The percentage of utilisation of ANC among students is higher (73.7 percent) than that of farmers (67.5 percent) and the others (71.4 percent). As such, the economic status as well as the first birth order seemed to influence the ANC utilisation. The previous history of bad health and complicacy during pregnancy and delivery also influence the mother for the utilisation of ANC. The results of field data indicates that there is a positive relationship between the complication during pregnancy or previous delivery with the utilisation of ANC where 83.8 percent of the mother who suffered from any health problems during pregnancy received ANC compared to 63.9 percent without any health problems. Similarly, mother who had experienced complication during delivery are found to access ANC (82.4 percent) compared to 66.2 percent without complications. As such, the health issues and delivery complicacy appears to be one major determinant of utilisation of ANC.

Table 5.13: Factors associated with the use of ANC

Characteristics of mother		Whether receive ANC?	
		Yes (N=193)	No (N=86)
Mothers age at last birth	15-19 Years	61.9	38.1
	20-29 Years	71.4	28.6
	30-39 Years	66.1	33.9
	40 And Above	33.3	66.7
Mother's level of education	No Education	52.5	47.5
	Primary	72.0	28.0
	Middle	74.4	25.6
	Secondary	65.2	34.8
	Higher Secondary	78.6	21.4
	Degree and Above	90.0	10.0
Distance from the nearest health facility	0-5 kms	70.1	29.9
	6-10 kms	65.5	34.5

Birth order	1st	81.0	19.0
	2nd - 3rd	68.4	31.6
	More than Three	57.7	42.3
During your pervious pregnancy did you suffer from any health problems?	No	63.9	36.1
	Yes	83.8	16.2
Mother's occupation	Farmer	67.5	32.5
	Services	100.0	
	Student	73.7	26.3
	Others (Business, Labour...)	71.4	28.6
During delivery did you experience any problems?	No	66.2	33.8
	Yes	82.4	17.6

Source: Own computation from field data, 2014.

5.3.2 Factors Associated with Institutional Delivery

As pregnancy and delivery is considered a natural process, mother may not feel it necessary to deliver in the health institution. However, various factors influence the mother to deliver in health institution. Table 5.5, shows the various factors that influences this decision making process of the mothers. Factors like age of the mother during last birth and level of education is examined to study the influence on institutional delivery. Institutional delivery is higher among the age group 15-19 (47.6 percent) and the age group 40 and above (66.7 percent). The institutional delivery increased with the level of education. The percentage of mother with no education who had institutional delivery is 20.3 percent and 75.0 percent among mother who are graduates. However for the group secondary and higher secondary level of education it is 39.1 percent and 29.1 percent respectively.

There is a negative relationship between institutional delivery and distance from health centre. Mothers living in the villages where health facility are located within 0-5 kms (34.9 percent) delivered more in the health facility than those living in the remote villages ranging from 6-10 kms away from the health facility (28.6 percent).

Table 5.14: Factors associated with the use of Institutional delivery.

Characteristics of mother		Place of delivery	
		Health facility (N=93)	Home (N=186)
Mothers age at last birth	15-19 Years	47.6	52.4
	20-29 Years	30.1	69.9
	30-39 Years	37.3	62.7
	40 and Above	66.7	33.3
Mother's level of education	No Education	20.3	79.7
	Primary	26.0	74.0
	Middle	35.6	64.4
	Secondary	39.1	60.9
	Higher Secondary	21.4	78.6
	Degree and Above	75.0	25.0
Distance from the nearest health facility	0-5 kms	33.9	66.1
	6-10 kms	30.9	69.1
Birth order	1st	50.0	50.0
	2nd - 3rd	23.9	76.1
	More than Three	29.5	70.5
During your pervious pregnancy did you suffer from any health problems?	No	31.7	68.3
	Yes	37.8	62.2
Mother's occupation	Farmer	29.9	70.1
	Services	62.5	37.5
	Student	42.1	57.9
	Others (Business, Labour...)	52.4	47.6
During delivery did you experience any problems?	No	25.4	74.6
	Yes	68.6	31.4

Source: Own computation from field data, 2014.

Birth order of the mother is also considered to investigate its impact on the institutional delivery. The above data shows a negative relationship between institutional delivery and birth order. In first birth it is found that 50.0 percent of women delivered in health facility which decreased to 29.5 percent in birth order of more than three. Thus, birth order or the experience over the period of time also determines the utilisation of institutional delivery.

Mother's occupation is observed to effect institutional delivery. Data suggests that percentage of institutional delivery is highest among the women who are in services (62.5 percent) and lowest percentage amongst the farmers (29.5 percent). The percentage of institutional delivery among schooling mothers is 42.1 percent which is higher than the farmer.

In the case of institutional delivery, learning from previous pregnancy and health related complications influenced mother's decision. It is found that 37.8 percent of the mother who had health problems during pregnancy delivered more in the institution compared to 31.7 percent of those without complications. In the same way, it is also found that 68.6 percent of the mother who had complication during previous delivery had delivered in the health facility compared to 25.4 percent with no complications. A positive relationship between the bad health experience at the time of pregnancy and during delivery with that of institutional delivery can be found. Hence, it can be concluded that the utilisation of ANC and institutional delivery is associated with factors common to both ANC and institutional delivery. Therefore, factors which lead to the higher utilisation of ANC also lead to higher institutional delivery.

5.4 Barriers to the Utilisation of Antenatal Care and Institutional Delivery

Although the utilisation of maternal health care is reasonably good but still many could not access it. In this sub-section, the reasons for non-utilisation of maternal health care have been discussed briefly. In Table 5.16 the reasons for not going to ANC check-ups is shown. Majority of the respondents (23.9 percent) feel that it is not necessary for them to visit health care facilities for ANC checks-up. Absence of complications during pregnancy (21.6 percent) is another major barrier effecting the utilisation of ANC. It is also found that 14.8 percent feel shy and 3.4 percent of the mothers have no time for ANC visit.

Table 5.15: Barriers to utilisation of ANC

Barrier	Percentage
Not necessary	23.9
Feel shy	14.8
Health facility too far	3.4
No time to go	3.4
Absence of complications during pregnancy	21.6
Not responded properly	6.8
Others(lack of knowledge, not customary, cost too much, poor quality service)	26.1

Source: Own computation from field data, 2014.

Table 5.16 shows that absence of complication during previous delivery (17.8 percent), feeling not necessary (17.3 percent) and sudden onset of labour (16.2 percent) are the major stated reasons for non-facility delivery. Similar to ANC, 12.0 percent of the mothers feel shy to deliver in health facility. Further, 12.0 percent of women felt uncomfortable and shy to go to health facility for delivery. Other reasons such as the health facility too far (6.3 percent), poor quality of health services (6.8) are also reported. In addition, time constraints (3.4 percent) are also cited as the reason for non-institutional delivery.

Table 5.16: Barriers to the Institutional Delivery

Barrier	Percentage
Not necessary	17.3
Feel shy	12.0
Health facility too far	6.3
Sudden onset of labour	16.2
No time to go	3.7
Absence of complication during previous delivery	17.8
Not responded properly	2.1
Poor quality of health service	6.8
No medical facility	.5
Others (no transport, no delivery preparedness, etc...)	17.3

Source: Own computation from field data, 2014.

As far as post natal care is concerned, the major reason reported is the absence of complications after delivery (74.5 percent). Similar to ANC and institutional delivery, mothers do not feel necessary to access PNC (9.1 percent). This is shown in table 5.17.

Table 5.17: Barriers to the utilisation of PNC

Barrier	Percentage
Not necessary	9.1
Health facility too far	2.2
No time to go	1.7
Absence of complication	74.5
Others	12.6

Source: Own computation from field data, 2014.

5.5 Conclusions

In this chapter we have presented various issues relating to the utilisation of maternal health care where we have discussed the status, factors associated with the utilisation of maternal health care and the barriers that prevent women from utilising MHC. We have found that the status of utilisation of maternal health care differs within the component of maternal health care. We have also found that utilisation of maternal health care varies with the age, education, distance from the nearest health facility, birth order, previous pregnancy complication and occupation of the mothers.

Chapter - VI

Findings and Conclusion

This piece of research entitled **Status of Maternal Health Care Utilisation: A case study of Mebo Sub-Division** has been carried out to highlight the status, utilisation and response of mother towards the health care facilities available to them. This chapter tries to discuss the principal findings to meet the stated objectives to conclude the study.

Pregnancy is one most crucial periods for women during which health care services are essential. Early detection of pregnancy related complications helps reducing maternal fatalities. Good health of mother before and after child birth is essential for the growth of the child, family and society as a whole. The government of India has therefore, implemented various programmes related to women/ mother health care services during pregnancy. Provisions have been made to promote ANC, Institutional delivery and PNC through various programmes like RHC, JSY and JSSK. These schemes have been implemented in the study area, except JSSK. The utilisation of maternal health care and the barriers related to non-utilisation of it have been examined. The major findings of the study are:

6.1 Socio-Economic Profile

It is found that while the percentage of total sample who attended primary level of education was 28.86 percent, percentage of sample that attained degree or above level of education was only 6.83 percent.

It is also found that 37.52 percent of the total sample is engaged in farming and only 2.88 percent of the total sample is in government services. More than 20 percent of the population are school goer. In general, it is found that more than 60 percent of the total sample is engaged in various occupations and the rest comprises of children (0-4 yrs), old age and those who are not employed in any activities.

The highest percentage of land holdings falls in the semi-medium category (32.3 percent). It is also found that 3.6 percent of the sample population does not have any landholding. Paddy is found to be the most commonly grown crop in the study area. However, cash crops like ginger, orange, mustard etc. are also found to be grown in the region.

The age composition of population shows that more than 45 percent of total sample are in working age group (15-44 years) whereas only 1.7 percent of the total sample are in old age group (65-80+ yrs).

It is found that 41.87 percent are currently married and only 9.12 percent of the sample population are not married. It is also found that people followed different religion of their choice but Donyi polo (indigenous faith) is found to be the highest (68.5 percent). The percentage of population who practised Muslim is only 0.7 percent (lowest).

It is found that different types of livestock are owned and reared in the study area like cow, Mithun, buffalo, pig, goat and poultry. 85.1 percent of the household owned pig and 76.2 percent own poultry. The most sacred animal Mithun is found to be reared by only 10.3 percent of the total sample.

6.2 Mothers Characteristics

1. About 70.3 percent of the mothers are in the age group 20-29 years, it is only 21.1 percent for age group 30-39 years which further decreased to only 1.1 percent for the age group above 40. This may be due to increasing awareness as well as availability of options.

2. The study found that 32.3 percent of the mothers had studied upto 6-8 years of schooling. Those in the range of 13-17 years of education are only 7.2 percent. Thus, the number of educated mothers decreased as the years of schooling increased, except for group from 0 and 1-5 YOS. This may be because most of the women get married at the very young age without attaining higher degree.
3. About 82.8 percent of the mothers are engaged in agriculture, while 2.9 percent are in the government service sector while about 7.5 are engage in sector other than the above two. About 6.8 percent are students. This show the changing perception and growing importance of education even amongst rural women and the family support therein.

6.3 Status of the Utilisation of Maternal Health Care

1. It is found that 69.2 percent of the mothers have received ANC irrespective of socio-economic background which is far above the state average whereas 30.8 percent of the mother could not receive ANC. About 50 percent of those who received ANC could not receive the minimum recommended ANC check-ups (four times) under JSY scheme. Many reasons have contributed to the non-utilisation of ANC. But the major reasons reported are the absence of sickness/complications during pregnancy (21.6 percent) and perceptions of women towards this service, as 23.9 percent of them feel it not necessary. In addition, many of them feel it not customary and also cited time constraint (3.4 percent) as one of the factor for the non utilisation of it.
2. It is found that status of institutional delivery is low in the study area (33.3 percent). The reasons for this are because of lack of delivery preparedness and sudden onset of labour (16.2 percent). In fact, 17.8 percent of the mothers do not feel it important or necessary to deliver in an institution. In addition, no complication during previous delivery is reported to be the one of the major reasons for low institutional

delivery (17.8 percent). The low delivery is also due to the fact that women feel shy to deliver at the health facility (12 percent). The home delivery is very high (66.7 percent) and majority of the delivery is conducted by traditional birth attendant (22.9 percent). These people are well experienced in conducting delivery though they are not trained. This resulted in high home delivery. It has also been found that the cash incentive provided by the government through JSY scheme could not attract much for the institutional delivery as only 21.2 percent of the mothers are JSY beneficiary.

3. The percentage of mother who utilised PNC is only about 17.2 percent. The most significant reasons reported for non utilisation of PNC are the absence of complications after delivery (74.5 percent). In addition, 9.1 percent of the mothers did not feel it necessary to go for PNC check-ups.

6.4 Factors Associated with the Utilisation of Maternal Health Care

1. It is found that relationship between the variables associated with the utilisation of ANC and institutional delivery are quite similar. While there is an increasing trend of utilisation of ANC between teenage and age group of 20-29 years, it decreased in age group above this. This may be because of unplanned or unintended pregnancy among teenage mothers, as they feel shy to go to hospital for check-ups. The utilisation of ANC is found to be highest in the age group of 20-29 years age group. This may be because women are more mature and most of them get married in this age group. Also this may be due to the fact that this age group is the prime child bearing age. In contrast, institutional delivery is lowest in this age group. This may be because with the increase in the child birth order the mother may not feel it necessary to deliver in health facility. In addition, the complication during delivery is likely to be less in this age group. Additionally, the utilisation of ANC decreases after

20-29 years which may be because the mother may feel that she has got enough experience and knows how to take care of herself. As a result, she feels reluctant to go for ANC. But the institutional delivery increases after 20-29 years which may be because of increasing delivery complication. Therefore, they prefer to deliver in health facility. Thus, the percentage of number of institutional delivery is highest in the age group above 40.

2. The utilisation of maternal health care is found to be influenced by maternal education. Nevertheless, the effect of education is not constant across all educational levels, nor is it the same in different components of maternal health care services. For instance, in case of ANC, it decreases in the secondary level of education. Similarly, among the mothers who have acquired higher secondary level of education, institutional delivery is less. However, after these fluctuations it goes on increasing. This is due to the reasons that with the increase in the level of education mother have more knowledge about health care and pregnancy related complications. In addition, education imparts feeling of self-worth and self-confidence which are critical in bringing about changes in health-related behaviour. Therefore, with the increase in the level of education the utilisation of maternal health care services increases.

3. There is a negative relationship between distance from the health facility and the utilisation of maternal health care services. Mothers living nearer to the health facility access more ANC than those living farther. The reason behind this may be because greater the distance greater the cost and time associated with it. Therefore, mothers with poor economic background cannot afford the cost of transportation and also bulk of the mother being farmers do not have time to go to health facility.

4. In relation to cost associated with the utilisation of maternal health care, it is found that mother's occupation also

determines the use of maternal health care. Mothers who are farmers are found to consume less of maternal health care services than that of those who are in services and others. Hence, the employment status is found to determine the use of maternal health care. This may be because of the fact that going to health facility is not free from cost. Although efforts have been made by the government to provide free medical care and incentive for institutional delivery, it does not meet the extra expenditure. Hence, a woman with higher occupational status is more likely to use maternal health care.

5. Birth order is found to be negatively associated with the utilisation of maternal health care. Because of the perceived risk associated with the first birth order, women seek more maternal health care. Thus, utilisation of maternal health care is higher in first birth order. With the increase in birth order, utilisation of maternal health care decrease. Such might be due to the fact that expectant mothers feel that she is already experienced to take care of the subsequent pregnancies. This may possibly be explained by the fact that women at higher birth orders may have had no difficulty during the previous births or that as the number of children increases in the household women has less time and greater responsibilities that may interfere with going to a health facility for delivery. Hence, she may not feel it necessary to go again and again to receive health care services for subsequent pregnancies.

6. The study reveals that previous history of a complication during pregnancy, delivery or post-delivery influences utilisation of maternal health care services. The more complications and health problems mother faced during pregnancy or previous delivery the more she utilised maternal health care Thus, there is a positive relationship between the previous complications during pregnancy and delivery and utilisation of maternal health care.

6.5 Barriers Associated with the Utilisation of Maternal Health Care

1. It is found that mothers perception towards the health care services are the most important barriers to the utilisation of MHC. It is found that 23.8 percent, 17.3 percent and 9.1 percent of the mothers feel not necessary to avail ANC, institutional delivery and post natal care respectively.
2. It is observed that until and unless no complications arises 21. 6 percent, 17.8 percent, 74.5 percent of the mothers do not like to avail ANC, deliver in institution and avail PNC respectively.
3. It is found that 14.8 percent of the mothers do not go for ANC as they feel shy. Similarly, 12.0 percent feel shy to deliver in health facility.
4. In addition to the above three points the study has also found many factors like health facility too far, no time to go, poor quality of health services, no medical facility, no transportation etc for non-utilisation for MHC.

6.6 Discussion

The descriptive and cross-tabulation analysis shows that various factors like mothers, age, educational level, distance from the health facility, occupation, birth order and the previous history of a complication influence the utilisation of maternal health care. The result in Table 5.5 and Table 5.6 shows that the maternal health care utilisation increase as the level of education increases. This finding is in line with the DLHS-3 (2007-08) report for Arunachal Pradesh and the study made in India where maternal education is found to be strongly associated with the utilisation of maternal health care (Gokhale et al; 2002, Jat et al; 2011). This finding suggests that higher level of education should be encouraged and interventions to educate girls and keep them from dropping out of school are thus critical to implement.

The results of this analysis show that younger women received more ANC than older women. But this is reverse in case of institutional delivery where older women deliver more in the institution. The result shows that child birth order emerge to influence the utilisation of these services. This result is in conformity with the findings of Singh et al (2012) and Jat et.al (2011) where the utilisation of maternal health care is higher among the women with the first order child birth than with those who had previous experiences of childbirth. To counter this complacency, reproductive health programmes must incorporate health education components that impart information about continued risks involved with delivering in the absence of trained assistance even though a woman may not have faced complications in the past.

As expected occupational status also emerge as a factor that influence the utilisation of these services. The higher occupational status is associated with higher utilisation of the services. This corroborates the findings of Shah, Bélanger, (2011) where women employed were found to utilise more of maternal health care. The result of this study shows that factor like distance from health facility exert as a significant influence on the utilisation of maternal health care services. Women living more nearer to the health facility utilised more of maternal health care than those living farther from the health facility. This finding is line with the findings of various studies in rural India (Sharan et.al; 2005, Kesterton et.al; 2010). The reasons for this case could be that transportation is unavailable. Even if women could get transportation, women could not bear the cost along with the accommodation cost that they might face to give birth in a distant health facility. This finding suggests that the effective working of ASHA will boost up the utilisation of these services. However this must be supplemented with the availability of emergency transport and referral services, since skilled attendants at home may be unable to deal with emergencies and unanticipated complications.

Past experiences of mother influence the utilisation of maternal health services. Mother who had previous bad experience of pregnancy and during delivery uses more of maternal health care. This finding is similar with the findings of Bhatia et. al. (2014). Approximately 18.3 percent and 26.5 percent of the mother had experienced problem during delivery and suffered from health problems during pregnancy. Such women are much more likely to seek an institutional delivery than problem-free women. This is an important finding because it implies that women make an appropriate response to pregnancy related complications.

6.7 Prescription

Health is an important factor that contributes to human wellbeing and economic growth. Maternal health care services are provided in the health facility. With the development of the health services in the state and implementation of various flagships programme by the government, mother's awareness about the basic health care services available to them during pregnancy has increased. However, in some of the rural areas perception of the utilisation of maternal health care is still in an embryo stage. The utilisation of maternal health care services in Mebo sub-division is reasonably good but its utilisation differs within the components of maternal health care. Where utilisation of ANC is high but it is low in institutional delivery and postnatal.

Numerous studies have found the influence of mother's age, education, occupations, birth order, previous history of pregnancy and delivery to the utilisation of maternal health care services. This research also confirms these findings. The low coverage of institutional delivery was due to the fact that women felt not necessary to deliver in an institution or because they were not ill during their labour or was not aware of the seriousness of the complications that they might face in delivery. Women did not consider Post natal care as important because of the absence of sickness and complications during delivery. Many of them don't go to the hospital if they don't have disease/ complications. This is not encouraging as it prevents the early detection of delivery related complications. Therefore, there is a need to advocate the importance of using maternal health care, so as to increase people's awareness of the benefits of such services to women's health. Lastly from the programmatic point of view, the conclusions reached in this research reinforce the call for continued investments in female education, which are indispensable to increase utilisation of maternal health care services. This research also confirms that, while the mechanisms of influence vary across different villages, education per se exerts a dominating influence. Nevertheless, public policies should not focus on education alone, as there are other factors, such as perception of women, access to health facilities, which affect health-care utilisation. Hence, improving access to health facilities should go hand in hand with educating women. By and large there is a need of proper counselling and educating women about the importance of registering with an ANM early for antenatal care, early detection of complications during pregnancy and promptly seeking care, and about the importance of giving birth in a health facility.

6.8 Future Research Agenda

The following points have been kept as future research agenda:

1. Since in the present study no econometric analysis is done, it can be done in future research.
2. Role of ASHA and Anganwadi worker in promoting maternal health care services.
3. The effectiveness of JSY in promoting maternal health care services.

Bibliography

Park, K. (2009). *Preventive and Social Science Medicine*. (20th edition). M/s Banardsidas Bhanot Publishers, Madhya Pradesh, India.

McGuire, Alistair, Henderson, John, & Mooney, Gavin (2005). *The economics of health care an introductory text, ISBN 0-415-06586-0* (Print Edition).

Abdul, Salam, & Siddiqui, S.A. (2006). Socio economic inequalities in use of delivery care services in India. *Journal of Obstet Gynecol India, 56 (2)*, 123-127.

Akum, Francis Abugri (2013). A qualitative study on factors contributing to low institutional child delivery rates in northern Ghana: The Case of Bawku Municipality. *Journal of Community Medical Health Education*, doi.org/10.4172/2161-0711.1000236.

Arthur, Eric (2012). Implications for maternal healthcare utilisation in Ghana. *Health economics review, 2(14).*

Asp, Gustav, Pettersson, Karen Odberg, Sandberg Jacob, Kabakyenga Jerome, & Agardh, Annette (2014). Associations between mass media exposure and birth preparedness among women in south western Uganda: A community-based survey. *Glob Health Action 2014, 7: 22904.* doi.org/10.3402/gha.v7.22904.

Becker, Stan, Peters, David, H., Gray, Ronald, H., Gultiano, Connie, & Bhatiaa, Jagdish C. and John Clelandb (1995). Determinants of maternal care in a region of South India. *Health Transition Review, 5*, 127 – 142.

Birmeta, Kidist, Yohannes Dibaba and Desalegn Woldeyohannes (2013). Determinants of maternal health care utilisation in Holeta town, central Ethiopia, *BMC Health Services Research.*

Bloom, Shelah, S., Wypij David & Gupta, Monica Das (2001). Dimension of Women's Autonomy and the Influence on Maternal Health Care Utilisation in North Indian City. *Demography, 38(1)*, 67-68.

Chakraborty, Nitai, Islam, Ataharul M., Chowdhury, Rafiqul Islam, Bari, Wasimul, & Hanum, Akhter Halida (2003). Determinants of the use of maternal health services in rural Bangladesh. *Health promotion international,18 (4).*

Chiang Chifa, Labeeb, Shokria Adly, Higuchi,Michiyo, Mohamed, Asmaa Ghareds, & Aoyama, Atsuko (2013). Barriers to the use of basic health services among women in rural southern Egypt (Upper Egypt). *Nagoya J. Med. Sci. 75*, 225 -231.

Chimankar, Digambar, A., & Saho, Harihar (2011). Factors Influencing The Utilisation Of Maternal Health Care Services In Uttarakhand. *Ethno Med, 5(3)*, 209-216.

Conrad, J.K., Hollenbach, K.A., Fullerton, J.T., & Feigelson, H.S. (1998). Use of prenatal services by Hispanic women in San Diego County a comparison of urban and rural setting. *Journal of Nurse-Midwifery 43(2)*, 90-96.

Erlindawati, Champikul, J, Isanarug, S (2008). Factors related to the utilisation of ANC services among pregnant women at health centres in Acwh Beasar District, Nanggroe Aceh Darussalam Province, Indonesia. *Journal of Public Health and Development vol 6(2).*

Exavery, Tanzania Amon, Almamy Malick Kante, Mustafa Njozi, Kassimu Tani1, Henry V Doctor, Ahmed Hingora and James F Phillips (2014). Access to institutional delivery care and reasons for home delivery in three districts of Tanzania. *International Journal for Equity in Health*, http://www.equityhealthj.com

Garg, Rajesh, Shyamsunder, Deepti, Tejbir Singh and Padda Avtar Singh (2010). Study on delivery practices among women in rural Punjab. *Health and Population: Perspectives and Issues, 33 (1)*, 23-33.

Gokhale, Medha, K., Rao, Shobha, S., & Garole, Varsha, R. (2002). Infant Mortality in India: Use of Maternal and Child Health Services in Relation to Literacy Status. *Journal of Health Population Nutrition, 20(2),* 138-147.

Jat, Tej Ram Nawing, & Sebastian, Miguel San (2011). Factors affecting the use of maternal health services in Madhya Pradesh state of India: A Multilevel Analysis. *International Journal for Equity in Health.*

Jena, S.K., Mahajan, P.B., & Bhatia, V. (2013). Status of institutional delivery in the state of odisha. *The Health Agenda, 1 (3)*, 49-56.

Laishram, Jalina, Thounaojam, Usha Devi, Panmei, Jina, Mukhia, Salona, & Lausharam, H. Sanayaima Devi (2013). Knowledge and practice of antenatal care in an urban area in India. *Indian Medical Gazzette, March 2013*, 101-106.

Mamatha, K.G., & Dr. Thimmaiah Navitha (2014). Impact of Janani Suraksha Yojana on institutional delivery and infant mortality rate in Karnataka. *International Journal of Research in Social Sciences, 4 (3)*, 444-454.

Manna, Prabir Kumar, & Dennassis De, & Ghosh, Debidas (2011). "Knowledge, attitude and practices for antenatal care and delivery of the mothers of Tea Garden in Jalpaiguri and Darjeeling Districts, West Bengal", *National Journal Of Community Medicine, 2(1).*

Matsumura, Masaki & Bina Gubhaju (2001). Women's status, household structure and the utilisation of maternal health services in Nepal. *Asia-Pacific Population Journal, 16 (1)*, 23-39.

Olayinka, Onasoga A., Achi, Osaji Teresa, Amos, Alade O. & Chiedu, Egbuniwe Michel (2014). Awareness and barriers to utilisation of maternal health care services among reproductive women in Amassoma Community, Bayelsa State. *International Journal of Nursing and Midwifery. 6(1)*, 10-15.

Priyanka Dixit "Improving Safe Childbirth in India" Population Reference Bureau Inform. Empower. Advance.

Shah, Reena, & Belanger Daniel (2011). Socio-economic correlates of utilisation of maternal health services by tribal women in India, *Canadian Studies in Population, 38(1), 83-98.*

Srivastava, Anand Kumar (2013). Factors associated with the preference for delivery at the government hospitals in rural areas of Lucknow district in Uttar Pradesh, *Indian Journal of Public Health, 57(4)*, 269-271.

Stekelenburg, J., Mukelabai Kyanamina, S., Wolffers, I., & Van, Roosmalen, J. (2004). Waiting too long: low use of maternal health services in Kalabo, Zambia. *Tropical Medicine and International Health 9(3*), 390–398.

Thind, Amarnand, Mohani, Amir, Banerjee, Kaberi, & Hagigi, Fred. (2012). Where to deliver? Analysis of choice of delivery location from a national survey in India, *BMC Public Health Journal Of Applied Medical Science, 1*, 93-116.

Varma, Deepthi, S., Khan, M.E., & Hazra, Avishek (2010). Increasing institutional delivery and access to emergency obstetric care services in rural Uttar Pradesh. *The Journal of Family Welfare* 56, *Special Issue.*

Wado, Yohannes Dibaba, Afework, Mesganaw Fantahun, &Michelle J Hindin (2013). Unintended pregnancies and the use of maternal health services in South Western Ethiopia. *BMC International Health and Human Rights 13:36.*

Worku, Awoke, Muhammed, Jemal, & Abeje, Gedefaw (2013). Institutional delivery service utilisation in Woldia, Ethiopia. *Science Journal of Public Health, 1(1),* 18-23.

Yared, Mekonnen & Mekonnen, & Asnaketch (2002). Utilisation of maternal health care services in Ethiopia, Ethiopian Health and Nutrition Research Institute, Addis Ababa, Ethiopia.

Anna Jallow, (2007). *Why are there low institutional delivery rates in the Gambia? Women's opinion*, (M. Phil Dissertation), University of Oslo.

Govindasamy, Pavalavalli, &Ramesh, B.M. (1997). *Maternal Education and the Utilisation of Maternal and Child Health Services in India, National Family Health Survey Subject Reports Number 5.*

Luis Pina Rebelo (2011). *The economics of health and health care: Assessing health determinants and impacts on an aging population* (Doctoral Thesis), Portuguese Catholic University.

Selma, J. Mushkin (1958). *Toward a Definition of Health Economies, Public Health Reports 73*(9).

Senapaty, Sagarika B.A., (2011). *Determinants of Utilisation of Reproductive Health Care Services in India: Involving Men in Maternal Health* (Master Thesis), Georgetown University, Washington, DC.

Yalem Tsegay Assfaw (2010). *Determinants of Antenatal Care, Institutional Delivery and Skilled Birth Attendant Utilisation in Samre Saharti District, Tigray, Ethiopia,* (Master Thesis), Umea International School of Public Health Department of Public Health and Clinical Medicine Epidemiology and Global Health, Umea University Sweden.

Desai, Sonalde, Lijuan, Wu, & Joshi, B.L. (2006). Utilisation of Maternal Health Care Services in India: Understanding the Regional Differences. India Human Development Survey Working Paper No. 1.

Ghosh, Sancheeta (2010). Increasing Trend in Caesarean Section Delivery in India: Role of Medicalisation of Maternal Health, working paper 236, ISBN 81-7791-192-9 © 2010, Copyright Reserved, the Institute for Social and Economic Change, Bangalore.

Kumar, Santosh, Dansereau, Emily, Murray, Chris (2014). Working Paper No. 14-05, SHSU Economics & Intl. Business, "Does Distance Matter for Institutional Delivery in Rural India"?

Shariff, Abusaleh, Singh, Geeta (2002). Determinants of Maternal Health Care Utilisation in India: Evidence from a Recent Household Survey Working Paper Series No. 85 *National Council of Applied Economic Research*, ISBN 81-85877-89-0

SRS government of India, 2006. Retrieved from http://censusindia.gov.in/vital_statistics/SRS-reports.html

State of the world's children, UNICEF 2009. Retrieved from www.unicef.org/sowc09/report/report.php

District level household survey 2012-13. Retrieved from https://nrhm-mis.nic.in/.../dlhs-4.aspx

National family health survey 3 2005-06. Retrieved from www.rchiips.org/nfhs/nfhs3.shtml

Online sources

http:// www.en.m.wikipedia.org/wiki/maternal_health

http:// www.un.org/millenniumgoals/maternal.shtml

http:// www.en.m.wikipedia.org/wiki/health_economics

http:// www.mohfw.nic.in

http:// www.nrhmarunachal.gov.in

http:// www.jstor.org

http:// www.censusindia.gov.in

Index

S

T

U

V

W

Y